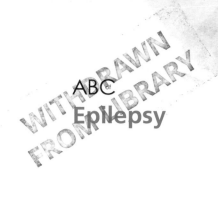

ABC of
Epilepsy

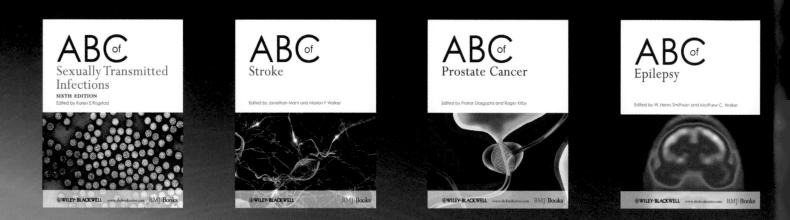

ABC of

Epilepsy

W. Henry Smithson

General Practitioner and Acting Head, Academic Unit of Primary Medical Care, Medical School
University of Sheffield, Sheffield, UK

Matthew C. Walker

Professor of Neurology, UCL Institute of Neurology
University College London and National Hospital for Neurology and Neurosurgery
London, UK

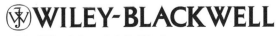

WILEY-BLACKWELL

A John Wiley & Sons, Ltd., Publication

BMJ|Books

This edition first published 2012 © 2012 by Blackwell Publishing Ltd.

Blackwell Publishing was acquired by John Wiley & Sons in February 2007. Blackwell's publishing program has been merged with Wiley's global Scientific, Technical and Medical business to form Wiley-Blackwell.

Registered office: John Wiley & Sons Ltd, The Atrium, Southern Gate, Chichester, West Sussex, PO19 8SQ, UK

Editorial offices: 9600 Garsington Road, Oxford, OX4 2DQ, UK

The Atrium, Southern Gate, Chichester, West Sussex, PO19 8SQ, UK

111 River Street, Hoboken, NJ 07030-5774, USA

For details of our global editorial offices, for customer services and for information about how to apply for permission to reuse the copyright material in this book please see our website at www.wiley.com/wiley-blackwell

Library of Congress Cataloging-in-Publication Data
ABC of epilepsy / edited by W. Henry Smithson and Matthew Walker. – 1st ed.
p.; cm. – (ABC series)
Includes bibliographical references and index.
ISBN 978-1-4443-3398-5 (pbk. : alk. paper)
I. Smithson, Henry. II. Walker, M. C. (Matthew Charles) III. Series: ABC series (Malden, Mass.)
[DNLM: 1.Epilepsy. WL 385]
616.85′3 – dc23

2011045228

A catalogue record for this book is available from the British Library.

Wiley also publishes its books in a variety of electronic formats. Some content that appears in print may not be available in electronic books.

Set in 9.25/12 Minion by Laserwords Private Limited, Chennai, India

Printed and bound in Singapore by Ho Printing Singapore Pte Ltd

1   2012

Contents

Contributors

Jan Bagshaw
Clinical Nurse Specialist, Community Epilepsy Services, Rochdale, UK

Colin D. Ferrie
Consultant Paediatric Neurologist, Leeds General Infirmary, Leeds, UK

Alice Hanscomb
Independent Trainer and Leadership Consultant, Director of Hanscomb Training & Consultancy, High Wycombe, UK

Mike P. Kerr
Professor of Learning Disability Psychiatry, Cardiff University; Welsh Centre for Learning Disabilities, Cardiff, UK

W. Henry Smithson
General Practitioner and Acting Head, Academic Unit of Primary Medical Care, Medical School, University of Sheffield, Sheffield, UK

Matthew C. Walker
Professor of Neurology, UCL Institute of Neurology, University College London and National Hospital for Neurology and Neurosurgery, London, UK

Foreword

Twenty years ago my partner, a young barrister, telephoned to say he was in hospital following a seizure whilst driving. Four months later he was seen by a neurologist, diagnosed and advised to take medication. Two months later he was discharged back to his GP, but died three months later suddenly and unexpectedly in his sleep. At no point was any information given about epilepsy or SUDEP (sudden unexpected death in epilepsy), and no one offered a helpline. Research and recognized good practice has advanced in leaps and bounds since my first encounter with epilepsy, and the editors, Henry and Matthew, are two of a small number of doctors who have made this happen.

I am honoured to write this foreword and must congratulate the editors and contributors on this wonderful book. Readers of this book will not only benefit from the expertise of researchers who are clinical leaders in the field, but will gain from the insight of professionals who have improved the lives of people with epilepsy and their families.

Epilepsy is the most serious common neurological condition. The impact of the epilepsies, however, remains underestimated. Epilepsy represents more than recurrence of seizures because it is associated with significant co-morbidities. Mortality rates have increased over the last 20 years when mortality rates have fallen across other conditions. In the UK, 70% of the population with epilepsy could be seizure free with optimal treatment, but only 52% achieve freedom from seizures.

This book is essential reading for any professional likely to come across epilepsy in their day-to-day practice.

Jane Hanna OBE
Director, Epilepsy Bereaved

Preface

The purpose of this addition to the ABC series is to provide a source of up-to-date information to enhance and broaden the management of a complex and challenging condition. Most current epilepsy texts have taken a predominantly biomedical perspective aimed at the specialist, but of less relevance to generalists involved in the management of people with epilepsy. We have addressed this gap by providing a practical approach to care throughout the patient pathway.

As a first step, it is critical to ensure that the diagnosis is correct and complete. Drug treatment should then be matched to the type of epilepsy and to the patient. However, there are other treatment modalities, and it is important to identify which people are suitable for these. Most importantly, the condition should be reviewed in a timely and supportive way. Epilepsy management is not just related to seizures, but encompasses numerous psychosocial challenges, which are often neglected. Patients need to be fully informed so that they can share in management decisions with clinicians to ease the burden of living with the condition.

This book is aimed at non-specialist physicians, general practitioners, practice and community nurses, clinicians in Accident and Emergency departments, doctors and nurses in training and those involved with the social aspects of care which is so important to many of those with epilepsy.

The editors have substantial experience in different aspects of care: one is an academic general practitioner with an interest in the condition who chaired the first NICE guideline group and was foundation chair of the UK International League against Epilepsy GP Society, and the other an academic neurologist with an international reputation in the field of translational epilepsy research and the management of people with drug resistant epilepsy.

The editors would like to record their thanks for expert contributions from other epilepsy specialists, epilepsy nurses and the voluntary sector. Thanks are also due to the National Institute for Health and Clinical Excellence for allowing us to use NICE Guideline CG20 as a resource that underpins much of this book.

Lastly we would like to thank Adam Gilbert (Commissioning Editor) and Kate Newell (Senior Development Editor) at Wiley Blackwell for their guidance and patience in the conception and delivery of this book.

W. Henry Smithson
Matthew C. Walker

CHAPTER 1

What is Epilepsy? Incidence, Prevalence and Aetiology

W. Henry Smithson[1] and Matthew C. Walker[2]

[1]Academic Unit of Primary Medical Care, Medical School, University of Sheffield, Sheffield, UK
[2]UCL Institute of Neurology, University College London and National Hospital for Neurology and Neurosurgery, London, UK

OVERVIEW

- Epilepsy is not a single condition but a term to describe a tendency to have recurrent unprovoked seizures
- It is the commonest serious neurological condition with an incidence of about 50 cases per 100 000 per year and prevalence estimated at 5–10 cases per 1000
- About 50% of cases have no identifiable cause, but the majority of new cases in adults is symptomatic and so investigations are needed to identify the underlying cause

---

Epilepsy is not one entity but more a fascinating group of conditions with many different manifestations depending on the part of the brain that is affected, the age of the individual, any underlying cause and the way that seizure activity spreads. It is one of the oldest recorded medical conditions. The first known written reference to it is in a Babylonian cuneiform dating back more than 3000 years, and epilepsy was considered a form of possession by a demon or departed spirit. Five hundred years later the same concept is present in Greek texts; indeed the word 'epilepsy' derives from the Greek for 'to possess' or 'to take hold of'. The Ancient Greeks considered that only the gods could knock someone unconscious, make their body thrash around uncontrollably, and afterwards bring them around with no apparent ill effects. Even today, seizures can be frightening to see, and lead to unnecessary prejudice and misunderstanding.

What is epilepsy?

An epileptic seizure is a clinically discernible event, which results from the synchronous and excessive discharge of a group of neurons in the cerebral cortex. The manifestation of a seizure depends on where in the brain it starts and how far and fast it spreads. Epileptic seizures usually have a sudden onset, spread in a matter of seconds or minutes and, in most instances, are brief. The seizure can be divided into a prodrome (the occasional recognition that a seizure will occur, sometime hours or days

beforehand), the seizure, which may include an aura (symptoms present at the beginning of a seizure), and lastly the post-ictal state (a period after the seizure during which the patient is usually confused). The mechanisms underlying seizure initiation and spread are still poorly understood, but involve the aberrant synchronisation of excitatory neurons, abnormal neuronal firing (e.g. burst firing) and a failure of inhibition. Seizures can therefore result from the ingestion of or withdrawal from drugs that affect neuronal activity (e.g. mefloquine, alcohol, benzodiazepines).

It is important to distinguish between seizures and epilepsy. Epilepsy is the tendency to have recurrent, unprovoked seizures. Seizures can result from specific precipitants such as fever in young children; soon after stroke; metabolic disturbances, for example hypoglycaemia; drug abuse/withdrawal; or acute head injury. These seizures are termed acute symptomatic seizures. Following such seizures, the chance of an unprovoked seizure is usually quite low and so the person would not be considered as having epilepsy. Similarly a single seizure is not usually considered sufficient to make a diagnosis of epilepsy. To make a diagnosis of epilepsy, there has to be a likelihood of having recurrent, unprovoked seizures. The seizure risk should be assessed when we are considering starting treatment, allowing someone to drive a car, fly a plane etc.

The tendency to have recurrent, unprovoked seizures results from alterations in brain excitability either as a result of genetic or environmental factors (or a combination of both). Epilepsy can therefore result from a number of underlying causes, and is thus best considered a symptom of an underlying brain disorder. The difficulties in attaching a threshold to the diagnosis of epilepsy have led to difficulties in epidemiological studies. For example, if someone is treated with antiepileptic drugs (AEDs) for a couple of seizures but has been seizure free for 10 years, would you consider them as having epilepsy?

Epidemiology

Given the variability in the definition of epilepsy, the incidence in the UK has been estimated to be approximately 50 cases per 100 000 people per year. No consistent national or racial differences have been found. However, the incidence is higher in low-income countries (probably due to the increased incidence of infective brain diseases), and in rural communities. The incidence of epilepsy has

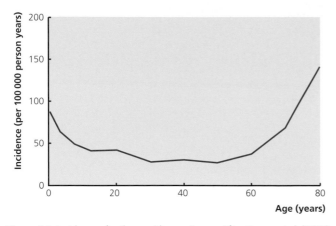

Figure 1.1 Incidence of epilepsy with age. *Source*: After Hauser *et al.* (1993).

a bimodal distribution with a peak in the first two decades of life (epilepsy secondary to genetic and congenital aetiologies) and a second peak in later life, over 60 years of age, due to late seizures after stroke and tumours (Figure 1.1). The incidence in children is decreasing, possibly due to better perinatal care, whilst the incidence in the elderly is increasing, possibly due to better survival of people following strokes.

Most prevalence studies of active epilepsy have found rates between 5 and 10 per 1000 persons in the population, regardless of location. Lifetime prevalence rates are much higher, and it is estimated that 2–5% of the population at age 70 years will have had epileptic seizures at some point in their lives (Figure 1.2); this is slightly higher in men than women. Epilepsy is more common in certain populations such as people with cerebral palsy and people with autism and/or learning difficulties.

The aetiology of epilepsy

Epilepsy is a symptom of an underlying brain disorder. It can present many years after a brain insult (such as perinatal hypoxia, brain injury etc.). Indeed, it is not uncommon for people with a brain injury in childhood to present with epilepsy in their twenties. This is termed remote symptomatic epilepsy. In approximately 40–50% of cases, although suspected, no known cause is found. With the advent of more advanced neuroimaging, this number is dwindling.

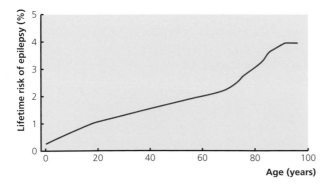

Figure 1.2 Cumulative prevalence of epilepsy. *Source*: After Hesdorffer *et al.* (2011).

The range of causation varies with age, and geographical location. The commonest acquired causes in young infants are perinatal hypoxia/asphyxia, perinatal intracranial trauma, metabolic disturbances, congenital malformations of the brain, and infection. In young children and adolescents, idiopathic (genetically determined) epilepsies account for the majority of seizure disorders. Adult epilepsies can result from initial causation in childhood but, in young adults, alcohol and head injury are amongst the commonest causes. In older adults, brain tumours are responsible for epilepsy in one-third of patients between the ages of 30 and 50 years, and cerebrovascular disease is the commonest cause of those over 50 years. In developing countries, parasitic disorders such as cysticercosis and malaria are important causes.

The range of recognisable aetiologies has changed with the advent of modern imaging, as subtle structural abnormalities such as hippocampal sclerosis and malformations of cortical development (dysplasia) are increasingly detected. Most epilepsies starting in adult life are symptomatic, and investigations to detect the underlying aetiology are mandatory.

Idiopathic (genetically determined) epilepsies constitute the majority of childhood epilepsies. These epilepsies are mostly polygenic and so confer only a moderately increased chance of offspring developing epilepsy – the first-degree relative of someone with idiopathic epilepsy is three-times more likely than the general population to develop epilepsy.

In addition to genetically determined conditions that have seizures as their main clinical expression, there are a large number of inherited disorders such as tuberous sclerosis and neurofibromatosis, in which epileptic seizures form only a part of the syndrome. Similarly there are other rare, inherited, degenerative brain disorders and inborn errors of metabolism that have seizures as part of the syndrome, such as mitochondrial disease, Tay–Sachs disease, phenylketonuria, porphyria and neuronal ceroid lipofuscinosis.

Prognosis

The prognosis of epilepsy depends upon a number of factors such as cause, age and genetic background. Our present treatments do not seem to have any impact on the natural history of epilepsy, but only treat the symptom – seizures. Nevertheless, for many people epilepsy is a transient condition. More than 70% of all people with epilepsy have their condition completely controlled with AEDs, and two-thirds of those will be able to stop medication without a recurrence of their seizures. However, 20–30% prove resistant to AED treatment and, for some, epilepsy surgery offers the best hope for a cure.

Chronic epilepsy has a significant social as well as medical impact on the individual. People with chronic epilepsy have an increased mortality rate, resulting from accidents, suicide and sudden unexpected death in epilepsy (SUDEP). SUDEP occurs in less than 0.1% of people with epilepsy per year. However, in those with refractory epilepsy, the risks of SUDEP may be as high as 0.5–1% per year. In addition to SUDEP, there is an increased risk of accidents such as drowning (19-times the risk of that in the general population) and, inexplicably, death from other causes such as heart disease and chest infections. People with chronic epilepsy have an increased risk of psychiatric co-morbidities, in particular depression, but also psychosis. Chronic epilepsy also has significant social implications, as people with continued seizures have a higher incidence of unemployment, problems with relationships and continued social stigma. Living with the condition is discussed in Chapter 9.

References

Hauser WA, Annegers JF, Kurland LT. Incidence of epilepsy and unprovoked seizures in Rochester, Minnesota: 1935–1984. *Epilepsia* 1993; **34**(3): 453–68.

Hesdorffer DC, Logroscino G, Benn EK, Katri N, Cascino G, Hauser WA. Estimating risk for developing epilepsy: a population-based study in Rochester, Minnesota. *Neurology* 2011; **76**(1): 23–7.

Further reading

Alarcon G, Nashef L, Cross H, Nightingale J, Richardson S. *Epilepsy*. Oxford Specialist Handbooks in Neurology. Oxford University Press, 2008.

Altrup U, Elger CE, Reuber M. Epilepsy Explained: A Book for People Who Want to Know More about Epilepsy. Medicine Explained Publishing, 2005.

Hart YM, Sander JW. *Epilepsy Questions and Answers*, 2nd edn. Merit publishing, 2008.

Hopkins A, Shorvon S. Definitions and epidemiology of epilepsy, in *Epilepsy*, 2nd edn (eds Hopkins A, Shrovon S, Cascino G). Chapman and Hall, 1995, pp. 1–24.

CHAPTER 2

Describing and Classifying the Condition

Colin D. Ferrie[1] and Matthew C. Walker[2]

[1]Leeds General Infirmary, Leeds, UK
[2]UCL Institute of Neurology, University College London and National Hospital for Neurology and Neurosurgery, London, UK

OVERVIEW

- The clinical manifestation of a seizure depends upon where in the brain it starts, and how far and fast it spreads

- Seizures are divided into two broad categories: those originating from a localised cortical area are classified as partial (focal) seizures (60% of cases), and those characterised by initial synchronous discharges over both hemispheres are classified as generalised seizures (40% of cases)

- An epilepsy syndrome consists of a combination of clinical, seizure and electroencephalograph (EEG) characteristics that make up a distinct entity

- Diagnosis of an epilepsy syndrome has implications for prognosis and management. However, diagnosis of a particular syndrome does not imply a single cause: many are known to have multiple aetiologies

---

The classification of epilepsy

While epilepsy is best considered a symptom of an underlying brain disorder, we can classify someone's epilepsy by aetiology, but this tells us very little about the clinical expression of the seizures, about the prognosis and about the expected findings on EEG. This information is contained within the classification of seizures and epilepsy. There is an accepted international classification of seizures and epilepsy that is at present under revision. However, the basic concepts will be preserved. The present International League against Epilepsy classification (Table 2.1) has a number of limitations, and is to some extent out of date in that it does not account for recent advances in genetics and neuroimaging.

Classification of seizures

The clinical manifestation of a seizure depends upon where in the brain it starts, and how far and fast it spreads. Seizures are divided into two broad categories: those originating from a localised cortical area are classified as partial (focal) seizures, and those characterised

ABC of Epilepsy, First Edition.
Edited by W. Henry Smithson and Matthew C. Walker.
© 2012 Blackwell Publishing Ltd. Published 2012 by Blackwell Publishing Ltd.

by initial synchronous discharges over both hemispheres are classified as generalised seizures. Seizures can sometimes, however, be difficult to classify. This is especially so with tonic–clonic seizures in adults, which can begin as a focal seizure that rapidly and extensively spreads, or which can begin simultaneously in both hemispheres (i.e. as a generalised seizure).

Partial (focal) seizures

Sixty percent of partial seizures originate in the temporal lobes (Figure 2.1), with the remainder usually beginning in the frontal lobes. Seizures originating in the parietal or occipital regions are relatively rare. Partial seizures are subdivided into three groups: simple partial, complex partial, and partial with secondary generalisation.

Simple partial seizures are focal seizures in which consciousness is fully preserved. They are usually brief, stereotypical and intense, and their manifestation depends upon where the seizure begins. Common symptoms in temporal lobe epilepsy include: déjà vu, 'butterflies', fear, illusions and hallucinations (auditory, olfactory and gustatory) and complex visual hallucinations. In frontal lobe epilepsies, there can be focal jerking that can spread as a 'Jacksonian March', more complex motor posturing, a difficult-to-describe feeling in the head, and forced thinking. In occipital lobe epilepsy, there can be simple visual hallucination, usually coloured blobs in one part of the visual field. With parietal lobe epilepsies there can be focal sensory phenomena such as tingling that is sometimes painful, somatic illusions such as distortion of mouth or limb, or even sensations of vertigo. Not unusually, the symptoms experienced during simple partial seizures can occur in people without epilepsy (e.g. déjà vu), but in epilepsy the occurrence is usually more frequent, more intense and often associated with other seizures in which consciousness is disrupted.

Complex partial seizures are focal seizures with impairment of consciousness. They can begin as a simple partial seizure (in this instance the simple partial seizure is often termed the 'aura'), or the person may have alteration of consciousness from the onset. In temporal lobe epilepsy, there may be motor arrest followed typically by chewing, lip smacking and swallowing (oroalimentary automatisms), and then fiddling with the hands (limb automatisms). Frontal lobe epilepsies can have more complex movements associated with them such as odd posturing ('fencing

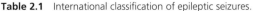

Table 2.1 International classification of epileptic seizures.

I Partial seizures
 A. Simple partial seizures
  1. With motor signs
   a. Focal motor without march
   b. Focal motor with march (Jacksonian)
   c. Versive
   d. Postural
   e. Phonatory
  2. With somatosensory or special-sensory symptoms
   a. Somatosensory
   b. Visual
   c. Auditory
   d. Olfactory
   e. Gustatory
   f. Vertiginous
  3. With autonomic symptoms or signs
  4. With psychic symptoms
   a. Dysphasia
   b. Dysmnesic
   c. Cognitive
   d. Affective
   e. Illusions
   f. Structured hallucinations
 B. Complex partial seizures
  1. Simple partial seizures at onset, followed by impairment of consciousness
   a. With simple partial features
   b. With automatisms
  2. With impairment of consciousness at onset
   a. With impairment of consciousness only
   b. With automatisms
 C. Partial seizures evolving to secondarily generalised seizures
  1. Simple partial seizures evolving to generalised seizures
  2. Complex partial seizures evolving to generalised seizures
  3. Simple partial seizures evolving to complex partial seizures evolving to generalised seizures
II Generalised seizures
 A. Absence seizures
  1. Typical absence seizures
   a. Impairment of consciousness only
   b. With mild clonic components
   c. With atonic components
   d. With tonic components
   e. With automatisms
   f. With autonomic components
  2. Atypical absence seizures
 B. Myoclonic seizures
 C. Clonic seizures
 D. Tonic seizures
 E. Tonic–clonic seizures
 F. Atonic seizures

Source: Adapted from Commission on Classification and Terminology of the International League Against Epilepsy (1981).

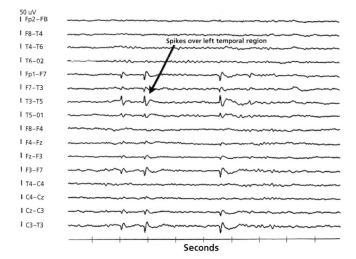

Figure 2.1 Interictal EEG with spikes over the left temporal lobe typical of temporal lobe epilepsy.

Secondarily generalised seizures are partial seizures, in which the epileptic discharge spreads to both cerebral hemispheres, so that a tonic–clonic seizure (convulsion) ensues. The patient may experience and recollect an aura, but this is not always the case if the seizure spreads rapidly.

Generalised seizures

The commonest of these are the tonic–clonic seizure and absence seizures, but there are also rarer seizure types that we will discuss.

Generalised tonic–clonic seizures (GTCS; often termed convulsions) usually occur without warning, although sometimes they can be preceded by increasing frequency of another generalised seizure type, such as myoclonic jerks or absences.

Initially the person is tonic (stiff) and may cry out (the 'epileptic cry'). The person will fall and may bite the side of the tongue as the jaw clenches. The person may also become cyanosed at this point. Clonic movements then begin, usually predominantly in the upper limbs. These are coordinated regular jerks that eventually slow and stop, at which point incontinence can occur. Most convulsions last less than 2 minutes. There is then a post-ictal period characterised by sleepiness and confusion lasting up to 20 minutes, but it may take longer for people to get over the full effects of the seizure (including lethargy, muscle aches, headache and a severely bitten tongue).

Typical absence seizures almost always begin in childhood or adolescence. There is motor arrest and staring. On occasions there can be fluttering of the eyelids, swallowing, and flopping of the head. The attacks usually last a few seconds, can occur many times a day and may be unrecognized, leading to a delay in diagnosis. There is immediate recovery and no post-ictal phase. This seizure type is associated with a characteristic EEG of three-per-second generalised spike-and-wave discharges (Figure 2.2). Typical absences need to be differentiated from complex partial seizures, which can sometimes also present as blank spells. There are also atypical absences, which are usually part of more severe epilepsy syndromes associated with learning difficulties, such as the Lennox–Gastaut syndrome (see below). In these the EEG is different, with slower and more

posture'), large gestural movements such as pushing away, or rocking, as well as running, scissoring or cycling movements of the legs. These movements can look quite bizarre but typically they are stereotypical, and witnesses will say that the same movements are seen with every seizure (although their severity can vary). Complex partial seizures are brief, usually lasting less than a few minutes. After complex partial seizures, people are usually confused (disorientated) for a time and are amnesic as regards the event.

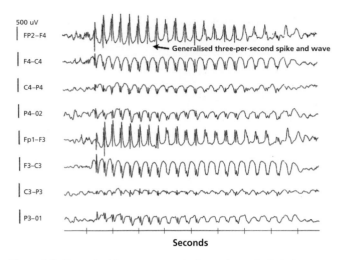

500 uV

FP2–F4

F4–C4

C4–P4

P4–02

Fp1–F3

F3–C3

C3–P3

P3–01

← Generalised three-per-second spike and wave

Seconds

Figure 2.2 Generalised three-per-second spike and wave typical of generalised absence epilepsy.

irregular spike-and-wave discharges. Also the onset and cessation of the seizure is less clear and there are often additional features such as changes in body tone.

Myoclonic seizures are sudden jerks that can involve a part of or the whole body. They commonly occur in the morning within a couple of hours of waking in idiopathic generalised epilepsies (see below). Although they usually occur in more benign epilepsy syndromes, they can rarely be associated with devastating epilepsies with cognitive and neurological decline – the progressive myoclonic epilepsies. Not all myoclonus is epileptic and can even be physiological, for example sleep starts (hypnic jerks).

Other generalised seizures consist of mainly atonic and tonic seizures. These are often termed 'drop attacks' and consist of sudden loss of body tone (atonic) or sudden increase in body tone (tonic), resulting in a fall. Recovery is generally rapid, notwithstanding any head injury. These seizures usually occur in more severe epilepsies with associated learning difficulties such as the Lennox–Gastaut syndrome.

Classification of epilepsy syndromes

An epilepsy syndrome consists of a combination of clinical, seizure and EEG characteristics that make up a distinct entity. Diagnosis of an epilepsy syndrome has implications for prognosis and management. However, diagnosis of a particular epilepsy syndrome does not necessarily imply a single aetiology: many epilepsy syndromes are known to have multiple aetiologies.

Some epilepsy syndromes are characterised by generalised seizures, others by focal seizures, and a few by both focal and generalised seizures. The first two of these can be considered generalised and focal epilepsy syndromes, respectively. Some epilepsy syndromes are always or nearly always idiopathic; others are always or nearly always symptomatic or probably symptomatic, but a number exist in idiopathic, probably symptomatic and symptomatic forms (e.g. West syndrome).

The term epileptic encephalopathy is used to denote epilepsies in which ongoing epileptic activity (either overt as clinical seizures or covert with ongoing epileptiform EEG discharges without obvious clinical seizures) gives rise to progressive (but potentially reversible) neurological dysfunction which can be manifested as learning and behavioural problems or occasionally as motor problems. Only a very small number of epilepsies follow this pattern.

Febrile seizures

Febrile seizures are the commonest type of epileptic seizure (occurring in 2–5% of the general population), but somewhat confusingly children with them are not considered to have epilepsy. This is because the seizures arise in the context of an external provoking factor (fever). They are epileptic seizures occurring in association with fever but without evidence of infection of the CNS, excluding those who have had previous non-febrile seizures or in whom there is a known cause of seizures. They usually occur between the ages of six months and six years. A family history is common. Most febrile seizures are GTCS, but other seizure types can be precipitated by fever, including tonic, clonic and myoclonic seizures. It is usual to classify febrile seizure as simple or complex. The latter implies that the seizure had focal features, was prolonged (usually defined as lasting 15 minutes or longer) or was repeated more than once during the same febrile illness.

In most children febrile seizures are self-limiting and benign. However, febrile status is the commonest cause of convulsive status epilepticus in children. One-third of children will experience one or more further febrile seizures. The risk of epilepsy is increased in children who have had a febrile seizure. By 25 years of age the risk of epilepsy is 7%. Risk factors for developing epilepsy after febrile seizures are family history of epilepsy, complex febrile seizures, and pre-existing neurodevelopmental problems. Many different types of epilepsy can follow febrile seizures. There is particular interest in the risk of temporal lobe epilepsy following prolonged febrile seizures.

Idiopathic generalised epilepsies

These are common forms of epilepsy occurring in childhood, adolescence and in adult life, and feature combinations of three seizure types: typical absences, myoclonic seizures and GTCS. In all of them a family history of epilepsy and of febrile seizures in infancy/early childhood is common. EEG shows generalised discharges of spike and wave or of spikes/multiple spikes, the latter being characteristic of syndromes with myoclonic seizures. Despite reports of linkage to a variety of chromosome regions and of specific mutations in individuals and families, their genetic basis is still unclear.

Childhood absence epilepsy is common in paediatric practice and usually starts between the ages of four and nine years. It is more common in girls than boys. It is characterised by typical absence seizures, usually lasting less than 20 seconds and occurring many times each day. The EEG is characterised by generalised 3-Hz spike-and-wave discharges. Response to appropriate medication is usually excellent, and most children become seizure free. The epilepsy commonly resolves, usually before age 12 years. However, a minority continue to have absences, and often develop GTCS.

Juvenile absence epilepsy is similar to childhood absence epilepsy, but is rarer and usually starts in later childhood or adolescence. The typical absence seizures occur less frequently, but GTCS are common and occasional myoclonic jerks may also occur.

Response to appropriate treatment is generally good, but the condition is likely to persist throughout adolescence and into adult life.

Juvenile myoclonic epilepsy is also common and probably under diagnosed. It usually begins between the ages of 10 and 18 years and has a genetic basis. The epilepsy consists of early morning and/or late-evening myoclonic jerks, tonic–clonic seizures (in most) and absences (in a third). At least 20% of patients with juvenile myoclonic epilepsy are photosensitive. Although the seizures can be well controlled with appropriate medication, the condition is usually lifelong.

(Benign) myoclonic epilepsy of infancy is rare, usually starting between six months and three years of age. The predominant, often sole, seizure type is myoclonic seizures occurring singly or in clusters. They may arise spontaneously or be provoked by noise or tactile stimuli. Remission commonly occurs between six months and five years after onset. A minority of children develop other seizure types and have educational problems.

Patients with **Doose syndrome** have myoclonic–astatic seizures; this starts in early childhood and is characterised by drop attacks caused by myoclonic seizures, atonic seizures (seizures characterised by a loss of muscle tone) or a combination of these seizure types (myoatonic seizures), and photically induced eyelid myoclonia with absences. Doose syndrome can also be classified as an epileptic encephalopathy (see later) because many children affected with it develop significant learning and behavioural problems.

Idiopathic and autosomal dominant focal epilepsies

The idiopathic focal epilepsies are very common forms of epilepsy occurring mainly in childhood. A family history of epilepsy and a history of preceding febrile seizures are common. Two examples of the commoner idiopathic focal epilepsies are benign Rolandic epilepsy and Panayiotopoulos syndrome. A number of rare focal epilepsy syndromes with autosomal dominant inheritance have been described. In some, causative gene mutations have been found, but these focal epilepsies are beyond the scope of this book.

Benign childhood epilepsy with centro-temporal spikes, which is also known as **benign Rolandic epilepsy**, usually starts in mid to late childhood and is probably the commonest type of new-onset epilepsy in otherwise normal children in this age group. The seizures are focal and characterised by tingling and numbness of the lips and tongue, and twitching at the corner of the mouth. Seizures may spread, leading to impairment of consciousness and/or hemiclonic or GTCS. A majority of seizures occur in sleep, during which spread may be very rapid, such that the initial focal onset is not apparent. The EEG characteristically shows so-called centro-temporal spikes. Seizure remission is expected within a few years, and certainly before the age of 16 years.

Panayiotopoulos syndrome is also common, usually occurring in children of about four to six years of age. The seizures are characterised by autonomic symptoms, particularly nausea, retching and vomiting, which usually begin in clear consciousness. Most seizures, however, progress with impairment of consciousness and sometimes hemiclonic and/or GTCS. Some seizures are mainly characterised by the child becoming flaccid and unresponsive. Characteristically the seizures are prolonged, often lasting over 30 minutes. A majority of the seizures occur in sleep and are very liable to be misdiagnosed. The EEG is characterised by multifocal spike-and-wave abnormalities. Total seizure count is usually low and remission is expected within a few years of onset.

Epileptic encephalopathies

These mostly occur in children. In the neonatal/early infantile period they include Ohtahara syndrome and early myoclonic encephalopathy. Both are very rare and are often associated with structural brain malformations and metabolic disorders, respectively.

West syndrome usually begins in the first year of life (peaking at three to nine months). The typical seizures are called epileptic or infantile spasms and consist of brief (up to a few seconds) episodes of contraction of truncal and limb muscles causing extension or flexion of the trunk and flexion or extension of the limbs. They may be quite subtle, particularly at onset. The seizures often occur in clusters, soon after awakening, on defecation or on feeding. The EEG usually shows a characteristic pattern termed hypsarrhythmia. An identifiable cause can be found in around 90% of patients. Structural brain abnormalities are common and can be genetic or acquired in origin. Tuberous sclerosis is the single commonest cause of West syndrome. Some chromosomal abnormalities, including Down syndrome, are associated with a greatly increased risk of West syndrome. Occasionally West syndrome arises as a consequence of metabolic disorders, which may require specific treatments.

Many children with West syndrome have developmental delay prior to onset of seizures. The onset of seizures is usually marked by developmental slowing, stagnation or regression, and many children with the disorder will ultimately be diagnosed with severe learning difficulties. Up to 20% eventually function within the normal range. This is more likely to be the case in those with idiopathic West syndrome. Epileptic spasms often subside after weeks, months or years. Some children remain seizure free but others develop other forms of epilepsy, including the Lennox–Gastaut syndrome.

Lennox–Gastaut syndrome is a rare epilepsy usually beginning in early–mid childhood and characterised by frequent seizures of multiple types including tonic and atonic seizures and atypical absences. Tonic–clonic, myoclonic and focal seizures may also occur. The tonic and atonic seizures often cause drop attacks. Episodes of convulsive and non-convulsive status epilepticus are common. The EEG is characterised by so-called slow (< 2.5 Hz) spike-and-wave discharges, and in-sleep runs of fast polyspike activity. The third component of the typical triad is learning difficulties (mild to severe), which may pre-date or follow the onset of the seizures, depending on the aetiology. As for West syndrome, which it often follows, it is usually symptomatic of various genetic and acquired structural brain disorders or metabolic disorders, but can arise de novo (idiopathic Lennox–Gastaut syndrome). The prognosis is poor. The syndrome can continue into adult life or evolve into a less well-defined epilepsy. Occasional patients do better, particularly those with idiopathic Lennox–Gastaut syndrome, those who are older at onset and those in whom a rapid response to treatment occurs.

Dravet syndrome (also known as severe myoclonic epilepsy of infancy) usually begins during the second half of the first year of life in a child who has been developing normally. Onset is typically with a febrile seizure, often prolonged with focal features, and may follow vaccination. Further similar seizures are likely over the next few months, some clearly febrile (but often low-grade fever), others during intercurrent illness without definite fever. Usually in the second or occasionally third year of life the picture changes, with multiple seizure types developing. These may include myoclonic seizures, atypical absences, GTCS and focal seizures. Episodes of non-convulsive status are common. Seizures often continue to be precipitated by fever and intercurrent illnesses. Accompanying the onset of this polymorphous epilepsy, developmental stagnation and even regression occurs and all affected children will eventually have severe learning difficulties, often with autistic behavioural problems. Motor problems, such as ataxia and spasticity, commonly develop. Eventually, often after some years, seizure frequency tends to reduce. The EEG is not particularly useful in the diagnosis, usually being normal early on. However, early photosensitivity is seen in a minority. Dravet syndrome is, in a majority, associated with identifiable mutations on the *SCN1A* gene which codes for a voltage-gated sodium channel.

Doose syndrome (see above under idiopathic generalised epilepsies) sometimes behaves as an epileptic encephalopathy, with around a half of those affected developing learning difficulties.

The **Landau–Kleffner syndrome** is a rare disorder usually occurring in previously normal children. It is characterised by a rather non-specific epilepsy (often mild) accompanied by regression in language and marked behavioural problems. Children developing it are often suspected of being deaf. It is usually accompanied by a characteristic EEG abnormality known as continuous spike and wave in slow wave sleep (CSWSS). The disorder is probably a consequence of ongoing epileptic activity in one or other superior temporal gyri. Similar problems can arise in children with other forms of epilepsy, with or without structural brain abnormalities, sometimes precipitated by AED medication.

Symptomatic/cryptogenic focal epilepsies

The symptomatic/cryptogenic focal epilepsies can occur at any age, and the seizure manifestation depends upon where in the cortex the seizure begins and how far and fast the seizure spreads.

References

Commission on Classification and Terminology of the International League Against Epilepsy. Proposal for revised clinical and electroencephalographic classification of epileptic seizures. *Epilepsia* 1981; **22**: 489–501.

Further reading

Forsgren L. Epidemiology and prognosis of epilepsy and its treatment, in *The Treatment of Epilepsy* (eds Shorvon S, Fish D, Perruca E, Dodson WE). Blackwell Science, 2004, pp. 21–42.

French JA, Delanty N (eds). *Therapeutic Strategies in Epilepsy*. Clinical Publishing, 2009.

Holmes GL. Classification of seizures and the epilepsies, in *The Comprehensive Evaluation and Treatment of Epilepsy* (eds Schachter SC, Schomer DL). Academic Press, 1997, pp. 1–36.

Hopkins A, Shorvon S. Definitions and epidemiology of epilepsy, in *Epilepsy*, 2nd edn (eds Hopkins A, Shrovon S, Cascino G). Chapman and Hall, 1995, pp. 1–24.

Nunes V, Neilson J, O'Flynn N, Calvert N, Kuntze S, Smithson H *et al. Clinical Guidelines and Evidence Review for Medicines Adherence: Involving Patients in Decisions about Prescribed Medicines and Supporting Adherence* (NICE Clinical Guideline CG76). National Collaborating Centre for Primary Care and Royal College of General Practitioners, 2009.

CHAPTER 3

Making the Diagnosis – Taking a History, Clinical Examination, Investigations

Jan Bagshaw[1], Matthew C. Walker[2], Colin D. Ferrie[3], Mike P. Kerr[4] and W. Henry Smithson[5]

[1]Community Epilepsy Services, Rochdale, UK
[2]UCL Institute of Neurology, University College London and National Hospital for Neurology and Neurosurgery, London, UK
[3]Leeds General Infirmary, Leeds, UK
[4]Welsh Centre for Learning Disabilities, Cardiff, UK
[5]Academic Unit of Primary Medical Care, Medical School, University of Sheffield, Sheffield, UK

OVERVIEW

- An accurate diagnosis of epilepsy depends on a detailed individual and witness history made by a specialist with an interest and expertise in the condition
- Misdiagnosis rates may be as high as 30%
- Clinical examination and investigations should be undertaken simply to support the history-based diagnosis and to rule out other co-morbidity
- Epilepsy in children may be part of a defined syndrome, and making a full syndromic diagnosis has prognostic and management implications
- People with learning disability pose a diagnostic challenge. The major traps are in behavioural outbursts, brief blank spells, nocturnal events and events that occur without convulsions. The diagnosis should be made by a specialist who may need videos or telemetry to assist diagnosis
- Older people have a high incidence of epilepsy (mainly focal in origin) and are at particular risk of injury. Epilepsy after stroke is common, and some medication can lower the seizure threshold

---

Making the diagnosis

The implications attached to making a diagnosis of epilepsy, both in adults and in children, are significant. The diagnosis affects health status, has a profound psychosocial impact and affects people's employment and education; so it is vital that the specialist is sensitive to the needs of the individual and their family and carers when communicating a diagnosis of epilepsy. However, making the diagnosis can be difficult.

Misdiagnosis is a frequent occurrence, particularly when the diagnosis is made by a non-specialist, resulting from either giving a label of epilepsy to people who do not have epileptic seizures or from not recognising epileptic events. Individuals misdiagnosed with epilepsy may experience social and financial deprivation as a

result of having the wrong diagnostic label and from side effects of AED medication, including the risk of unnecessary teratogenicity. Misdiagnosing epilepsy as a psychiatric disorder disadvantages the affected individuals not only with an incorrect diagnosis but also by the effects and risks of continuing seizure activity because appropriate AEDs are not used. In a small number of cases, individuals die prematurely because the correct diagnosis of epilepsy was not made, and a serious condition was neither diagnosed nor treated. It is therefore crucial that specialists involved in diagnosing epilepsy take great care to establish the correct diagnosis. The complete care pathway is summarised in Figure 3.1.

Taking a history

Differentiating between epileptic seizures and other causes of transient neurological disturbance depends on a detailed and clear description of the event. The affected individual may not be aware of the attack, and so establishing a correct diagnosis often depends on a witness account or a video of an event. The diagnosis should be made by a specialist with training and expertise in the condition, and an urgent referral should be made after the first episode (the National Institute for Health and Clinical Excellence (NICE) recommend being seen within two weeks).

There are no 'gold standard' investigations that clinicians can order to make the diagnosis. The place of investigations is discussed later, but is only to support a diagnosis made by taking a careful history.

When taking a history it is crucial to identify any spontaneous or otherwise unexplained paroxysmal symptoms. Symptoms include:

- sudden falls;
- involuntary jerky movements of limbs while awake;
- blank spells;
- unexplained urinary incontinence with loss of awareness, or in sleep;
- odd events occurring in sleep, e.g. falling out of bed, jerky movements or automatisms;
- episodes of confused behaviour with impaired awareness.

ABC of Epilepsy, First Edition.
Edited by W. Henry Smithson and Matthew C. Walker.
© 2012 Blackwell Publishing Ltd. Published 2012 by Blackwell Publishing Ltd.

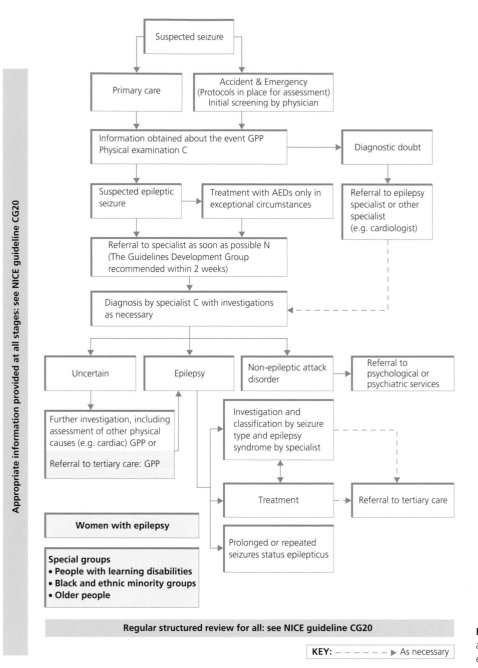

Figure 3.1 Summary NICE outline care algorithm for adults. *Source:* CG20; Stokes *et al.* (2004).

'Major events' such as a generalised convulsive seizure are relatively well known, but 'minor' seizures can have an equally profound effect on the individual and are often missed. Importantly, such minor events can also herald a more severe seizure.

It is important to enquire about transient and paroxysmal feelings that may be as a result of focal seizures, such as epigastric rising sensation, déjà vu, premonitions, fear, elation, depression, depersonalisation or derealisation, inability to understand or express language, loss of memory or disorientation, hallucinations (olfactory, gustatory, visual, auditory), focal motor or somatosensory deficit or positive symptoms like jerking or tingling.

Many such feelings can be experienced by people without epilepsy, but in epilepsy, they are often intense, unexpected, frequent and stereotypic.

The previous chapter describes how a complete diagnosis should include the type of epilepsy, classification of seizures and identification of any underlying causality. This is usually determined by the specialist. A community-based case-notes review revealed the variability and inaccuracy of epilepsy diagnosis in letters sent from specialist epilepsy clinics to general practitioners, and so accuracy of the diagnosis should be checked at each epilepsy review.

Clinical examination

It is good practice to perform a general clinical examination on patients presenting with new seizures. Patients expect a careful assessment and are reassured by this. It also gives the clinician an opportunity to find signs of an underlying cause such as evidence of stroke (common), cutaneous signs of tuberous sclerosis (rare), or evidence of an intracranial tumour in older people. A clinical examination can also exclude signs of other morbidity such as valvular disease, arrhythmia, raised intracranial pressure or carotid bruit.

Investigations

- Routine blood tests (plasma glucose, electrolytes, calcium) should be performed to rule out co-morbid conditions and to identify any underlying cause. Importantly, seizures can present for the first time in pregnancy. In children, blood and urine biochemistry investigations are not recommended routinely but will be appropriate in specific circumstances, as determined by an appropriate specialist.
- Neuroimaging should be used to identify structural abnormalities that cause certain epilepsies (Figure 3.2). Magnetic resonance imaging (MRI) scans should be obtained in all individuals with epileptic seizures unless there is a secure diagnosis of febrile seizures, one of the idiopathic generalised epilepsies, or of benign Rolandic epilepsy. Imaging is crucial in patients developing epilepsy under two years of age or, in adulthood, in patients with suggestive focal seizures on history, examination or EEG. Imaging should also be considered in patients with seizures refractory to first-line medication. MRI is the investigation of choice but computed tomography (CT) is acceptable if MRI is unavailable or contraindicated. In younger children who would require a general anaesthetic for an MRI, CT may also be appropriate. EEG should only be performed to support a diagnosis of epilepsy where the seizures are considered likely to be epileptic in origin. EEG should not be performed in patients with syncope or non-epileptic attack disorder (NEAD) because of the possibility

of a false positive result. EEG can be helpful in determining epilepsy syndrome or in classifying seizures, and can be useful in assessing risk of seizure recurrence if there is evidence of unequivocal epileptiform activity.
- Functional scanning: there is a range of increasingly sophisticated methods of assessing cerebral blood flow in regions of the brain, between and even during seizures, and to identify the cerebral areas that are responsible for cognitive processes. Such investigations can be of importance in pre-surgical assessment. Cerebral metabolites and neurotransmitters can also be investigated, but usually as part of clinical studies at tertiary centres.
- Measurement of serum prolactin level is not recommended for the diagnosis of epilepsy, as it may not rise in complex partial seizures and conversely can rise with syncope and even psychogenic attacks.
- Electrocardiogram (ECG) should be a standard investigation for most paroxysmal events, particularly convulsive seizures, to exclude arrhythmias and prolonged Q-T syndrome.

Common misdiagnoses

The four common differential diagnoses for seizures are syncope, psychogenic non-epileptic seizures, migraine and parasomnias. The important differentials in non-specialist practice are epilepsy, syncope and psychogenic events, and the key features are set out in Table 3.1. Syncope can be differentiated from seizures by situation, prodrome and nature of the attacks. Vasovagal attacks occur when standing or sitting and are often precipitated (e.g. by pain, fear etc.). They are usually preceded by a warning in which the patient feels dizzy, hot and nauseous. Before blacking out, the vision greys or becomes blurred and sound may appear distant. Pallor, profuse sweating and slumping are usually observed. Recovery of consciousness is usually rapid and any confusion is short lived. Occasionally, prominent autonomic symptoms can be present during a seizure, making diagnosis more challenging.

Psychogenic non-epileptic seizures (PNES; often termed dissociative seizures or pseudoseizures) are psychologically driven episodes over which the person has little conscious control (they are therefore distinct from malingering). A variety of semiology is possible, ranging from slumping (the classic 'swoon') to thrashing around. Injury can occur, and certain injuries such as carpet burns to the face are more common in such attacks than in epilepsy. Eyes held shut, long periods of apparent loss of consciousness, pelvic thrusting, thrashing and directed violence are all features of PNES. Overt psychiatric disease may not be present, and such attacks may be learnt stress reactions in people who have experienced bullying, torture, physical or sexual abuse.

Migraine is usually easy to differentiate from seizures. However, seizures originating in the occipital lobe may have a visual aura and a headache. The visual aura of seizures differs in that it is stereotypical (always affecting the same part of the visual field) and evolves rapidly and is present for a matter of minutes in contrast to the aura of migraine which usually lasts more than five minutes. Rarely, brainstem migraine (usually with brainstem symptoms such as diplopia and vertigo) can result in loss of consciousness. In addition, migraine aura can occur without headache (acephalgic migraine).

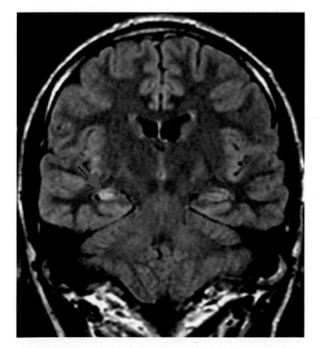

Figure 3.2 MRI showing hippocampal sclerosis.

Table 3.1 Differential diagnosis of epilepsy.

	Differential diagnosis		
	Epilepsy	**Syncope**	**Psychological causes**
Circumstance	Unpredictable Sleep or wake Occasionally precipitant	Upright Precipitant	Observed Often precipitant
Prodrome/aura	Stereotypical Brief Evolve	Presyncope Can be prolonged	Dissociation Autonomic features
Event	Stereotypical Brief Evolve	Pallor Variable semiology Brief (Non-coordinated jerking can be seen)	Slumping Eyes shut Thrashing Directed violence Waxes and wanes Prolonged
After the event	Confusion	Unwell	Tearful

Events at night can be difficult to diagnose because of a poor description of the event. Seizures usually occur many times throughout the night, and cluster. In contrast, parasomnias usually occur once or twice a night and are restricted to certain parts of the night. Non-rapid eye movement parasomnias are common in children but also affect 2% of adults. They mainly consist of sleep walking, night terrors and confusional arousals. They occur from deep sleep (usually during the first third of the night). Rapid eye movement sleep behavioural disorders are more common in the elderly and in men, and consist of dream enactment, usually towards the morning. In cases where the diagnosis is in doubt, video-EEG telemetry is necessary (even then, diagnosis of brief events at night can be difficult).

Diagnostic considerations in special groups

Learning Disability

It is a sensible precaution to be particularly precise in making a diagnosis of epilepsy in individuals with a learning disability. People with a learning disability make up a large proportion of the population of people with epilepsy, and their epilepsy is often severe, complicated and chronic. However this very over representation can contribute to misdiagnosis, as epilepsy can be expected to be present and clinical acumen may wane; an example of diagnostic overshadowing.

The core of epilepsy diagnosis in this group is the clinical history and recognition of behaviour that sound like seizures. The clinical history often comes from a third party, and episodic behavioural disturbance has a broader differential diagnosis. For the clinician the problem is not so great when an individual has a classical generalised tonic–clonic seizure. It is when events occur without convulsions that most problems occur. The major traps are in behavioural outbursts, brief blank spells and in nocturnal events.

Behavioural outburst should not be considered as having a basis in epilepsy without detailed specialist assessment, which will include videos and may include telemetry. Blank spells have a broad differential diagnosis including depression, and autonomic dysfunction in rare conditions such as Rett syndrome, and again need further assessment. Nocturnal events are often seizures.

A practical approach is to employ the same principles as in any other individual with a potential diagnosis of epilepsy, but to be particularly cautious of events without a convulsive element and to be very cautious of applying a diagnosis of epilepsy without having seen, at a minimum, a video of the event.

Older people

The diagnosis of epilepsy in older people may cause concern to the individual because of the memories of how epilepsy was viewed when they were younger as a difficult-to-control and stigmatising condition that was not uncommonly associated with brain damage and cognitive impairment. There may be continuing concern about the associated risk of injury particularly due to the prolonged post-ictal state common in older people.

The majority of seizures in the elderly are focal in origin, and the onset of primary generalised seizures is rare in this age group but can occur, especially on sudden withdrawal of benzodiazepines. Obtaining a witness history can be problematic and the clinician may have to rely on a third-party description of the post-ictal state. EEG investigation should be regarded with caution because of the increasing range of normal appearances in the older brain.

The differential diagnosis of transient impairment or loss of consciousness will include syncope, hypoglycaemia, transient ischaemic attacks or behavioural change due to organic brain disease.

An underlying cause should be sought and will include early (within one week) or late (more than one week) post-stroke seizures, myoclonic seizures associated with Alzheimer's disease or seizures caused by cerebral tumours. Cardiac arrhythmias and subdural haematoma should be excluded.

Seizure threshold can be lowered by certain drugs including prednisolone, insulin, oral hypoglycaemic agents, antibiotics, tricyclic antidepressants or lithium. Withdrawal from alcohol or benzodiazepines can also cause seizures in older people.

Children

In babies, infants and younger children it is not possible to obtain a description of the phenomena which can characterise epileptic seizures. Sometimes it is possible to make inferences from observed changes in behaviour. For example, the young child who suddenly looks terrified and runs to his mother before becoming unresponsive with automatisms may be experiencing a temporal lobe seizure. Considerable skill is needed to take a history from younger children who are verbal. However, the results can be very rewarding. Children as young as four may be able to describe the vivid visual hallucinations which characterise occipital lobe seizures. Children often have seizures at night when the eyewitness may be a sibling, or at school in front of their classmates or teacher. Trying to reconstruct a paroxysmal event from a third-party account is usually frustrating and frequently misleading. Attempts should be made to interview those who have witnessed attacks. Where teachers are concerned it can be helpful for the clinician to provide written advice as to what information is likely to be particularly useful should further attacks be witnessed.

The range of non-epileptic paroxysmal events which occur in children is age dependent and large, particularly in infancy. No one should attempt to diagnose epileptic seizures in children unless they are familiar with these other disorders. Some of these, such as breath holding attacks and reflex anoxic seizures, are very common. Homemade recordings of non-epileptic attacks (now usually made on mobile phones) are often available and are an invaluable aid to diagnosis.

Most described epilepsy syndromes are childhood disorders. Many are age dependent. A syndrome diagnosis is possible in a majority of children with epilepsy, but certainly not in all. Moreover, it may only be with the passage of time that a syndrome diagnosis can be made confidently. It is important not to 'force' children into a particular epilepsy syndrome diagnosis. This constitutes one type of epilepsy misdiagnosis.

Idiopathic forms of epilepsy are common in childhood, but an underlying cause for the epilepsy should be sought depending on the clinical features of the individual case. If an epilepsy syndrome diagnosis has been made this will help determine whether and what investigations are appropriate. An underlying cause for epilepsy is particularly likely in those under two years of age. NICE recommends such children are seen by a paediatric neurologist.

Metabolic investigations are unlikely to be informative unless there are specific markers suggesting that the seizures are symptomatic of one of these conditions. Genetic investigations, particularly chromosomal analysis, should be considered on the basis of the family history, examination findings (e.g. dysmorphic features) and co-morbidities, particularly learning difficulties.

Finally the diagnostic process is not complete until an appropriate assessment of co-morbidities and the effect of the seizures on the child's personal, family, school and social life has been made. The rate of learning difficulties and behavioural problems is much higher in children with epilepsy than in the general population and indeed higher than in children with most other chronic disorders.

References

Stokes T, Shaw EJ, Juarez-Garcia A, Camosso-Stefinovic J, Baker R. Appendix A: Differential diagnosis of epilepsy, in *Clinical Guidelines and Evidence Review for the Epilepsies: Diagnosis and Management in Adults and Children in Primary and Secondary Care* (NICE Clinical Guideline CG20). Royal College of General Practitioners, 2004.

Further reading

Hamandi K. Epilepsy, in *Brocklehurst's Textbook of Geriatric Medicine and Gerontology*, 7th edn (eds Fillit HM, Rockwood K, Woodhouse K). Saunders Elsevier, 2010, pp. 453–66.

Hopkins A. The causes of epilepsy, the risk factors for epilepsy and the precipitation of seizures, in *Epilepsy*, 2nd edn (eds Hopkins A, Shrovon S, Cascino G). Chapman and Hall, 1995, pp. 59–85.

Leach J-P, Lauder R, Nicholson A, Smith DF. Epilepsy in the UK: misdiagnosis, mistreatment and undertreatment? The Wrexham area epilepsy project. *Seizure* 2005; **14**: 514–20.

Nunes V, Neilson J, O'Flynn N, Calvert N, Kuntze S, Smithson H *et al*. *Clinical Guidelines and Evidence Review for Medicines Adherence: Involving Patients in Decisions about Prescribed Medicines and Supporting Adherence* (NICE Clinical Guideline CG76). National Collaborating Centre for Primary Care and Royal College of General Practitioners, 2009.

CHAPTER 4

Managing the Drug Treatment of Epilepsy

Colin D. Ferrie[1], Mike P. Kerr[2], W. Henry Smithson[3] and Matthew C. Walker[4]

[1]Leeds General Infirmary, Leeds, UK
[2]Welsh Centre for Learning Disabilities, Cardiff, UK
[3]Academic Unit of Primary Medical Care, Medical School, University of Sheffield, Sheffield, UK
[4]UCL Institute of Neurology, University College London and National Hospital for Neurology and Neurosurgery, London, UK

OVERVIEW

- Antiepileptic drug treatment is the commonest treatment for epilepsy, and the majority of patients can expect full seizure control

- Treatment should be individualised according to seizure classification, type of epilepsy, co-morbidity and the risk of future seizure

- Starting treatment should be decided between prescriber and patient, with monotherapy as the aim, to reduce the risks of teratogenicity and side effects. Patients therefore need information about the condition and their medication

- Any change in medication should be made slowly with a second drug allowed to reach effective levels prior to withdrawing the original drug. Consistency of formulation is advised

- Between 15 and 30% of patients may not take their medicine as prescribed

- Routine blood monitoring except for phenytoin is not recommended if the dose is stable, seizures are controlled and no side effects are noted except for phenytoin

- There are special considerations when treating people with a learning disability, or children

---

The majority of patients can achieve complete seizure control by taking antiepileptic drugs (AEDs). Antiepileptic drugs can be effective, but like all drugs acting on the CNS, cause side effects (see Table 4.1, adapted from Stokes *et al.* (2004)). AEDs do not 'cure' epilepsy; there is no evidence that they can influence the prognosis of the epilepsy. The decision to prescribe AEDs should be shared with the patient, who should be provided with information about the drug (including indications, side effects and licence status) and information about the condition including risks of not taking medication (see Chapter 9).

General principles

The AED treatment strategy should be individualised, taking account of the type of epilepsy, seizure classification, co-morbidity and co-medication, the individual's lifestyle and views about medicines.

The diagnosis of epilepsy needs to be critically reviewed if episodes continue despite an optimal dose of a first-line drug.

Changing the formulation of the drug is not advised, because of the variable bioavailability or pharmacokinetics between formulations that may result in reduced efficacy or increased side effects.

Treatment should be with a single drug wherever possible to reduce interactions and side effects (including teratogenicity). If the first AED is unsuccessful, then gradual transition to a second agent may be necessary. Start at a low dose and gradually increase the dose until seizure control is achieved or side effects are noticed – 'start low and go slow'.

Changing of an AED should be managed by a clinician with expertise, who will introduce the second drug while maintaining the dose of the first drug until reaching an optimal dose with the second agent. The dose of the first AED is then slowly reduced and withdrawn.

Combination therapy may be considered if monotherapy fails to control seizures, but if the combination does not lead to benefit, then consideration should be given to reverting to the most acceptable single-drug regimen.

The decision about drug treatment should be shared between prescriber and patient to optimise adherence to medicines. To do this, the patient will need information about the proposed drugs (Box 4.1).

Starting treatment

Antiepileptic drugs should only be introduced when a firm diagnosis of epilepsy has been made. Initiation should be by a specialist and with the agreement of the patient, after a full discussion of the benefits and risks of treatment.

One of the main considerations of whether to start treatment is the chance of seizure recurrence. After a single seizure, the recurrence rate is approximately 50% within two years, with most of this risk in the first three to six months. Where there is an identifiable and avoidable provoking factor the recurrence rates are lower. However, in the presence of cerebral palsy or a progressive neurological lesion (e.g. tumour), the recurrence rate is considerably higher. For the most part, treatment is not usually started after a single seizure except when a seizure is associated with a

---

ABC of Epilepsy, First Edition.
Edited by W. Henry Smithson and Matthew C. Walker.
© 2012 Blackwell Publishing Ltd. Published 2012 by Blackwell Publishing Ltd.

Box 4.1 **Information about medicines**

Patients need information, about their condition and possible treatments, for involvement in decision-making. The format and content should meet the needs of individual patients.

- Before you prescribe, offer patients (including inpatients) clear, relevant information. This will probably include, but should not be limited to:
  - what the medicine is, how to use it, and likely benefits and side effects
  - what to do if they miss a dose.
- Check patients have any information they wish before medicines are dispensed.
- Check patients have understood the information and discuss it with them, taking into account what they know and believe about the medicines.
- Do not assume that patient information leaflets (PILs) will meet all patients' needs. Address any concerns raised after reading PILs.
- Suggest where patients might find reliable information and support after the consultation (for example, websites).

Source: After Nunes *et al.* (2009).

neurological deficit present at birth, a seizure is associated with a clearly abnormal EEG (such as the presence of 3-Hz spike and wave), or a seizure occurs in the context of a progressive neurological disorder. Treatment approximately halves the risk of further seizures. There is no evidence that delaying treatment until the second seizure changes the prognosis of the epilepsy.

In contrast, two unprovoked seizures within a year carries a recurrence risk of over 80%, and treatment should be started unless there is significant uncertainty concerning diagnosis, or the seizure occurred in the setting of certain benign seizure syndromes (e.g. Rolandic epilepsy).

There is, at present, no evidence to indicate that prophylactic AED treatment, after head injury, febrile convulsions or neurosurgery, prevents the occurrence of epilepsy in the longer term (it may prevent the occurrence of acute seizures).

Continuing treatment

Continuing treatment should be decided by the specialist, and the patient should be given an individual agreed management plan that includes the indications of the chosen AED, the recommended dose, and what to do if seizures or side effects persist.

Once treatment is stable, repeat prescriptions may be obtained through general practice with usual medication and epilepsy review (Chapter 8).

Once a prescription has been given for the AED, clinicians should be aware that between 15 and 30% of patients may not take medicines as prescribed (non-adherence).

To reduce the rate of non-adherence (Nunes *et al.*, 2009), you need to understand the patients' concerns and beliefs about

treatment. You can improve your understanding of the patient's perspective by:

- asking patients what they know and believe about medicines before prescribing, and when reviewing;
- asking about general or specific concerns (such as side effects or dependence), and addressing these;
- bearing in mind that patients may wish to minimise their medicines and to discuss
  - what will happen if they don't take the medicine
  - non-pharmacological alternatives
  - reducing or stopping long-term medicines
  - fitting medicines into their routine
  - choosing between medicines.

Choosing an antiepileptic drug

This is the role of a specialist, and a guide to AED indications can be found in the updated NICE guideline. Ordinarily, lamotrigine and carbamazepine are the first-line AEDs of choice in partial epilepsy. The situation in generalised epilepsies is more complicated, because evidence indicates that valproate has the best efficacy, but because of its high teratogenic risk is not the treatment of choice in women of childbearing age (see Chapter 7).

Side effects are a major determinant in AED choice (see Table 4.1). People on long-term AED treatment are at increased risk of osteoporosis. All adults on AED treatment should, therefore, have vitamin D and calcium monitored every three to five years, and patients in higher risk groups should also have bone density measurements.

Randomised control trials of new AEDs usually compare their use as add-on treatment in drug resistant partial epilepsy compared to placebo, and there are no good trials comparing individual drugs. The choice of add-on medication, in those not seizure free with first-line therapies, therefore represents a significant clinical challenge.

Monitoring antiepileptic drug levels

Routine blood monitoring is not recommended if the dose is stable, seizures are controlled and no side effects are noted. The concentration range for an AED is a guide based on population data, and there are people who require a lesser level or can tolerate a higher level. Dosing should therefore be guided by clinical response. There is good evidence that increasing the dose of drugs in someone who is seizure free to achieve a 'therapeutic' level does not decrease the chance of subsequent seizures, but rather increases the chance of side effects.

There are certain circumstances where monitoring may be undertaken:

- detection of non-adherence or suspected toxicity
- adjustment of phenytoin dose
- managing pharmacokinetic interactions
- managing situations that affect drug levels, such as pregnancy or concomitant illness.

Table 4.1 Antiepileptic drug side effects.

Drug	Significant side effects include:
Acetazolamide	Some loss of appetite, depression, 'tingling' feeling in the extremities, polyuria, thirst, headache, dizziness, fatigue, irritability and occasional instances of drowsiness.
Carbamazepine[a]	Allergic skin reactions, including urticaria, which may be severe. Accommodation disorders, for example blurred vision, diplopia, ataxia and nausea. Particularly at the start of treatment, or if the initial dose is too high, certain types of adverse reaction occur very commonly or commonly.
Clobazam	Drowsiness has been reported. Tolerance may develop, especially during prolonged use.
Clonazepam	Somnolence and fatigue have been observed: such effects are usually transitory and disappear spontaneously as treatment continues or with dosage reduction. With certain forms of epilepsy, an increase in the frequency of seizures during long-term treatment is possible.
Eslicarbazepine	Very common side effects include dizziness and somnolence. Common side effects include nausea, double vision and rash.
Ethosuximide	Mild side effects, which are usually transient, may occur initially. These include headache, nausea and drowsiness. Other adverse reactions reported include weight loss and irritability.
Gabapentin	The most common possible side effects are somnolence and dizziness. A common side effect is fatigue. Headache has also been reported.
Lacosamide	The most common side effects are dizziness, headache, nausea and diplopia. Lacosamide can also prolong the P-R interval in the ECG and so should be used with caution in people with heart disease.
Lamotrigine	Skin rash, which generally appears within eight weeks of starting treatment and resolves on withdrawal. Adverse experiences reported include drowsiness, diplopia, dizziness, headache, insomnia, tiredness, fever (associated with a rash as part of a hypersensitivity syndrome) and agitation, confusion and hallucinations.
Levetiracetam	Most common reported undesirable effects include dizziness and somnolence. Other undesirable effects include irritability, insomnia, ataxia, tremor, headache and nausea.
Oxcarbazepine[a]	Very common undesirable effects include diplopia, headache and nausea. Common undesirable effects include skin rash, ataxia and confusion.
Phenobarbital[a]	Drowsiness, lethargy and mental depression.
Phenytoin[a]	Hypersensitivity reactions including skin rash. Common undesirable effects include drowsiness, ataxia and slurred speech, and these are usually dose related. Coarsening of facial features, gingival hyperplasia and hirsutism may occur rarely. Some haemopoetic complications have been reported including some anaemias (these usually respond to folic acid). Motor twitchings, dyskinesias (rare), tremor (rare), and mental confusion have all been observed.
Piracetam	Reported effects (incidence of between 1 and 3%) include weight increase, insomnia, somnolence, nervousness, depression and (incidence less than 1%) diarrhoea and rash.
Pregabalin	The most common side effects are dizziness and tiredness. Weight gain can also sometimes be troublesome.
Primidone[a]	Most common side effects include drowsiness and listlessness, but these generally occur only at the beginning of treatment. Other effects have been reported but are usually transient. On occasions, an idiosyncratic reaction may occur, which involves these symptoms in an acute and severe form necessitating withdrawal.
Retigabine	Very common side effects include fatigue, dizziness and somnolence. Rarely urinary retention can occur and so should be used in caution in high risk groups.
Rufinamide	Very common side effects include somnolence, headache, dizziness and nausea. Rash can also commonly occur.
Sodium valproate	Sedation and tremor have been reported occasionally. Transient hair loss, which may sometimes be dose related, has often been reported. Regrowth normally begins within six months. Increase in weight may also occur. Severe liver damage has been very rarely reported. Encephalopathy and pancreatitis may occur rarely. Also, hyperammonaemia without change in liver function tests may occur frequently and is usually transient. Blood dyscrasias may occur frequently, and the blood picture returns to normal when the drug is discontinued. Sodium valproate has been associated with amenorrhoea and irregular periods. Any menstrual problems should be reported to the general practitioner and neurologist. Sodium valproate is associated with a higher risk of fetal malformations if taken in pregnancy.
Tiagabine	Dizziness, tiredness, nervousness (non-specific), tremor, concentration difficulties and depressed mood.
Topiramate	Headache, somnolence, dizziness, paraesthesia and weight decrease. Increased risk of nephrolithiasis. Difficulty with memory and concentration/attention has been reported. Cases of eye reactions – secondary acute angle closure glaucoma presenting as painful red eye or acute myopia – have rarely been associated with topiramate occurring within one month of starting treatment.
Vigabatrin	Somnolence is very common, while nausea, agitation, aggression, irritability and depression are common. Psychosis has been reported as uncommon. Visual field defects have been reported in one in three people taking vigabatrin, with onset usually after months to years of treatment. Any person who has concerns about this should talk to their general practitioner and neurologist. Visual field tests should be performed every six months in patients on vigabatrin.
Zonisamide	Agitation, irritability, confusion, depression, poor muscle coordination, dizziness, poor memory, sleepiness, double vision, loss of appetite and decreased blood levels of bicarbonate have all been commonly reported with zonisamide. In addition, nephrolithiasis can occur in up to 1% of treated individuals.

[a]Hepatic-enzyme-inducing drug.
Source: Stokes *et al.* (2004).

Withdrawing antiepileptic drugs

This should only be done under specialist guidance with the agreement of the patient, after full discussion of the risks and benefits. All patients should be warned of the dangers of abrupt cessation and should be given advice about what to do if they forget a dose (usually to take the missed dose at the next opportunity).

Usually drug withdrawal is not considered unless someone has been at least two years seizure free. Overall, after two years of seizure freedom, the chance of seizure recurrence without AED withdrawal over the next two years is 20% and this climbs to 40% with AED withdrawal. The risk is dependent upon clinical circumstance and, the longer that someone has been seizure free, the greater the chance of successful AED withdrawal. If someone wishes to withdraw then they should be given up-to-date advice about driving regulations when withdrawing from AEDs, and it must be explained to them that, if they have a seizure, they will lose their driving licence and they will have to inform the DVLA.

Following the maxim 'start slow – go slow', any planned withdrawal should be conducted slowly over two or three months, withdrawing one agent at a time. Some drugs such as barbiturates or benzodiazepines must be withdrawn more slowly, perhaps over six months.

Patients should reverse the last dose change and seek urgent medical advice if seizures recur.

There are special considerations when treating people with a learning disability, or children.

Learning disability

When considering drug treatment for an individual with a learning disability, it is crucial to have specialist knowledge of the complex epilepsy syndromes associated with learning disability and epilepsy, and the ability to judge treatment outcome. Rare paediatric epilepsy syndromes such as Lennox–Gastaut and Dravet syndrome are over-represented in adults with a learning disability. These syndromes are characterised by a range of seizure types and a greater severity of epilepsy. In addition to these, people with a learning disability often have multiple seizure types. Such syndromes may need a specific approach to drug choice.

The biggest issue facing a clinician is managing treatment outcome. This again splits into two components: judging treatment success and assessing side effects.

When individuals have new epilepsy or few previous treatments, then seizure freedom should be the expected goal. However a large part of the population will have a more complex and refractory epilepsy. In this group in particular, an individual approach is paramount, with a broad approach to treatment success that should be individually based and can include: seizure freedom, seizure reduction, reduction of one seizure type such as drop attacks, reduced hospitalisation, reduced injury, and a greater number of seizure-free days.

Side effects are of great concern for all individuals with learning disability and epilepsy. When drugs are assessed in randomised control trials in people with a learning disability, the side effects seen are very much typical of those seen in the general population, and abnormal behaviour is not frequent. However, in a clinical setting, concerns about behavioural side effects are frequent. A holistic approach is needed as behaviour patterns are most often long standing, but can also reflect acute environmental change, physical or psychological disorder. Drug reduction is only recommended when these have been excluded, often by engaging with psychology and other services.

Children

Antiepileptic drug treatment is not recommended for febrile seizures and children with single or very infrequent seizures. The decision to start a child on antiepileptic drug treatment should usually be made by assessing how unpleasant/disruptive the seizures are to the child. In most situations the choice of AED and how it is used is similar to adult practice, with doses usually being calculated according to weight.

Antiepileptic drug treatment does not, in a large majority of patients, change the ultimate prognosis in terms of the likelihood of seizure remission, and treating with AEDs to avoid learning and behavioural problems is problematic given the neurobehavioural side effects of AEDs. An exception is the epileptic encephalopathies, in which rapid control of seizures may increase the likelihood of terminal remission and limit the development of learning and behavioural problems. Most clinicians consider AED treatment after a child has had two or three seizures. However, most only treat a minority of children diagnosed with benign Rolandic epilepsy and Panayiotopoulos syndrome with regular AEDs.

Some AEDs used in adult practice are not licensed for some or all children. The converse is also true in some cases. Concern about hepatic toxicity with sodium valproate somewhat limits its use in babies and infants. Vigabatrin, now very rarely used in adult practice because of retinal toxicity, is a drug of choice for infantile spasms and seizures in tuberous sclerosis, and ethosuximide is a drug of choice (along with sodium valproate) for childhood, but not juvenile, absence epilepsy. This is because it has specific activity against absences, but not GTCS. Steroids (prednisone orally and ACTH injections) are used to treat certain childhood epileptic encephalopathies, especially West syndrome.

Routine blood tests prior to and after starting AEDs in the hope of being able to avoid or detect early adverse effects, although often recommended by manufacturers, are not in practice predictive, and are discouraged by NICE. However, HLA testing of individuals of certain races, particularly those of Chinese origin, prior to treatment with carbamazepine in order to avoid Stevens–Johnson syndrome, should be considered. Routine blood level monitoring is generally used only with phenytoin.

References

Nunes V, Neilson J, O'Flynn N, Calvert N, Kuntze S, Smithson H *et al. Clinical Guidelines and Evidence Review for Medicines Adherence: Involving Patients in Decisions about Prescribed Medicines and Supporting Adherence* (NICE Clinical Guideline CG76). National Collaborating Centre for Primary Care and Royal College of General Practitioners, 2009.

Stokes T, Shaw EJ, Juarez-Garcia A, Camosso-Stefinovic J, Baker R. Appendix B: Pharmacological treatment, in *Clinical Guidelines and Evidence Review for the Epilepsies: Diagnosis and Management in Adults and Children in Primary and Secondary Care* (NICE Clinical Guideline CG20). Royal College of General Practitioners, 2004.

Further reading

Forsgren L. Epidemiology and prognosis of epilepsy and its treatment, in *The Treatment of Epilepsy* (eds Shorvon S, Fish D, Perruca E, Dodson WE). Blackwell Science, 2004, pp. 21–42.

Patsalos PN. *Anti-epileptic Drug Interactions – A Clinical Guide*. Clarius Press, 2005.

Patsalos PN, Bourgeois BFD. *The Epilepsy Prescriber's Guide to Antiepileptic Drugs*. Cambridge University Press, 2010.

Taylor MP. *Managing Epilepsy – A Clinical Handbook*. Blackwell Science, 2000.

A useful site for specific drugs can be found at www.medicines.org.uk/ guides/epilepsy.

CHAPTER 5

Non-drug Treatments Including Epilepsy Surgery

Colin D. Ferrie[1], W. Henry Smithson[2] and Matthew C. Walker[3]

[1]Leeds General Infirmary, Leeds, UK
[2]Academic Unit of Primary Medical Care, Medical School, University of Sheffield, Sheffield, UK
[3]UCL Institute of Neurology, University College London and National Hospital for Neurology and Neurosurgery, London, UK

> **OVERVIEW**
>
> - The impact of seizures can sometimes be reduced by non-drug treatment
> - Psychological interventions, vagal nerve stimulation, ketogenic diet and surgical resection are interventions that may be considered for some patients with refractory seizures, both to reduce seizure frequency and to address the low mood and poor self-esteem associated with epilepsy
> - Seventy percent of patients with operable structural abnormalities can be rendered seizure free after resective surgery, but appropriate selection of patients is crucial

While the majority of people with epilepsy can anticipate good seizure control with the correct antiepileptic drugs, about 30% of people continue to have seizures. This individual burden is exacerbated by a feeling of social stigma, fragmentary and sometimes ill-informed care from the health service and the challenge of overcoming the psychological impact of the condition.

Non-pharmacological treatment can be helpful to address these problems.

Epilepsy surgery

Epilepsy surgery in those with drug resistant temporal lobe epilepsy is one of the few surgical procedures that have been the subject of a randomised controlled trial compared against continued medical management. The study indicated that the chance of seizure freedom was sevenfold higher in the surgical group. Epilepsy surgery therefore often represents the best chance of seizure freedom in those resistant to antiepileptic drugs. Epilepsy surgery is more successful and has a greater psychosocial impact the earlier it is done in the course of the epilepsy. In view of this, it is generally recommended that those people with partial epilepsy that have tried therapy with at least two first-line antiepileptic drugs appropriate

for their epilepsy, at adequate doses, and who are not seizure free after two years, should be considered for epilepsy surgery. This is because the chance of becoming seizure free with continued drug management is only 10%. In contrast, approximately 70% of people will become seizure free with resective surgery (depending on lesion and brain area), and most will remain so over the longer term (10–20 years). Even in those for whom curative resective surgery is not possible, palliative surgery can reduce the severity and/or frequency of seizures. Epilepsy surgery should be carried out in specialist centres with access to a multidisciplinary team to assess and monitor the impact of surgery on cognition, memory and mood.

Psychological interventions

Epilepsy can be associated with depression and poor self-esteem. People may feel that the condition controls their lives, and yet there is evidence to show the benefits of regaining control over the condition and their lives. This can be aided by provision of information about the condition and regular individual review (Chapter 8).

There are a number of counselling styles, but all effective psychosocial interventions focus on current individual relevant problems, a clear structure or plan of treatment, and delivery based on an effective patient–practitioner relationship. The professional should adopt an open consulting style to encourage active listening, to allow the patient an opportunity to discuss their problems (National Collaborating Centre for Mental Health, 2009). We will describe person-centred counselling and cognitive behavioural therapy (CBT).

Person-centred counselling uses a flexible approach to let the individual come to decisions about what is best for them and how they want to change their lives. Counselling is available in a number of settings, with psychological therapies offered by practice-based counsellors in primary care, by psychology services managed by the Primary Care Trust or by specialist services in secondary care (Williams and Garland, 2002). Patients with NEAD may benefit from the specialist services of a neuropsychological counsellor.

Cognitive behavioural therapy is based on similar principles, but the approach is more goal focused and encourages people to change how they think (cognitive) and what they do (behaviour). The Royal College of Psychiatrists web page gives an excellent outline

---

ABC of Epilepsy, First Edition.
Edited by W. Henry Smithson and Matthew C. Walker.
© 2012 Blackwell Publishing Ltd. Published 2012 by Blackwell Publishing Ltd.

of the therapy, where detailed resources on CBT can be found and from where much of the information given here on psychological interventions and biofeedback has been taken (Blenkiron and Timms, 2011). CBT can be offered one to one, as a group, or using computerised programmes ('Fear Fighter' for people with phobias or panic attacks and 'Beating the Blues' for people with mild to moderate depression; Williams and Martinez, 2008). Unlike some of the other talking treatments, it focuses on the 'here and now' problems and difficulties. Instead of focusing on the causes of your distress or symptoms in the past, it looks for ways to improve your state of mind now. CBT is indicated in a number of conditions; for example anxiety, depression, certain phobias, eating disorders, obsessive-compulsive disorder and post-traumatic stress, as well as situations where there is anger or low self-esteem.

Cognitive behavioural therapy can break down seemingly overwhelming problems into manageable parts. When a situation occurs, we make a psychological assessment (our thoughts) that lead to emotions, actions and feelings. Psychiatrists describe how 'this vicious circle' can make one feel worse, and how CBT can help you break away from this circle of 'altered thinking, feelings and behaviour'.

These areas are interdependent, and the problem may be managed by thinking positively around each area to dispel unhelpful feelings. They suggest a useful acronym, 'Change View', to capture the elements of the therapy (Box 5.1).

Box 5.1 **Change View – 10 key facts about cognitive behavioural therapy**

Change: your thoughts and actions
Homework: practice makes perfect
Action: don't just talk, do!
Need: pinpoint the problem
Goals: move towards them
Evidence: shows CBT can work

View: events from another angle
I can do it: self-help approach
Experience: test out your beliefs
Write it down: to remember progress

Source: Adapted from Blenkiron and Timms (2011).

CBT can be effective but is not for everyone. It takes some time for the therapy to work and needs a significant time commitment. Patients may be able to access CBT through their general practitioner. The British Association for Behavioural and Cognitive Psychotherapies holds a register of accredited therapists, and there are self-help programmes available.

Biofeedback

An individual may be able to alter their mental and physical state through techniques of relaxation and being attuned to feedback from their bodies. There has been a keen debate about whether a person with epilepsy can stimulate an anticonvulsant EEG rhythm (the sensorimotor rhythm) and so reduce the frequency of seizures. There are some systems that use cranial sensors to measure the change in electrical activity. Neuro-biofeedback is the process of measuring and monitoring this activity, but gaining individual control involves a technically complex method that can be time consuming, and the enthusiasm for sensorimotor rhythm-based biofeedback has waned (Brown, (1995)). Current guidance recommends that psychological therapies may improve quality of life but should not be seen as an alternative to drug treatment and may not have an effect on seizure frequency.

Vagal nerve stimulation

Vagal nerve stimulation (VNS) is used to reduce seizures in patients with drug resistant epilepsy, and requires a surgically implanted mechanical stimulator (a *pulse generator*) placed subcutaneously on the chest wall with a wire leading to the left vagus nerve in the neck. The generator sends regular electrical stimulation to the nerve. The aim is to reduce the number and severity of seizures, and this is recommended for adults and children over 12 years of age with refractory generalised or partial seizures who are not suitable for surgical resection. VNS can reduce seizure frequency by 50% in about 25% of treated patients, and this reduction compares favourably with newer AEDs. The evidence in the NICE guidelines suggests that VNS remains effective in the long term, with a satisfactory safety profile. The stimulator can be boosted by passing a magnet over the device, and this is useful for patients with pre-ictal aura to prevent the development of a seizure. The effect of VNS is not immediate and some people find the effect on seizures can take up to two years. The stimulator is set for the individual and set at a low amplitude which is gradually increased over time. Commonly the stimulator is active for 30 seconds every 5 minutes both day and night. Side effects are only experienced while the stimulator is active and include discomfort in the throat, a cough, difficulty swallowing and a hoarse voice. One positive effect is that VNS can reduce the symptoms of depression, indeed refractory depression is another indication for use. As the stimulator is metallic, care should be taken if an MRI scan is being considered.

Ketogenic diet

The ketogenic diet was devised over 80 years ago when the treatment options for epilepsy were limited to barbiturates and bromides. It was found that induced ketonuria reduced seizures. Ketonuria is induced by a high fat, low carbohydrate, low protein diet to mimic the body's biochemical response to starvation. The classical ketogenic diet provides about 80% of calories as fat, predominantly long-chain fats such as butter and cream. The modified ketogenic diet makes use of medium-chain triglyceride (MCT) oil, which allows more carbohydrate to be given. The diet is complex and requires close co-operation between carers, clinicians and dieticians in order to obtain adequate ketonuria and avoid short and long-term adverse effects. There is good evidence of the efficacy of the ketogenic diet in reducing the frequency of seizures across a range of childhood epilepsies. It should be considered in children with drug resistant epilepsy who are not suitable for resective epilepsy surgery.

Access to specialist clinics with expertise in initiating and managing the diet is limited in the UK.

References

Blenkiron, P; Timms P (ed.). The Royal College of Psychiatrists: Cognitive Behavioural Therapy. Online leaflet produced by the RCPsych Public Education Editorial Board. Available at www.rcpsych.ac.uk/mentalhealthinfoforall/treatments/cbt.aspx (accessed August 2011).

Brown S. Other treatments for epilepsy, in *Epilepsy*, 2nd edn (eds Hopkins A, Shorvon S, Cascino G). Chapman and Hall, 1995, pp. 309–14.

National Collaborating Centre for Mental Health. *Depression: The NICE Guideline on the Treatment and Management of Depression in Adults. Updated Edition* (NICE Clinical Guideline CG90). The British Psychological Society and The Royal College of Psychiatrists, 2009.

Williams C, Garland A. A cognitive–behavioural therapy assessment model for use in everyday clinical practice. *Advances in Psychiatric Treatment* 2002; **8**:172–9. doi: 10.1192/apt.8.3.172

Williams C, Martinez R. Increasing access to CBT: stepped care and CBT: self-help models in practice. *Behavioural and Cognitive Psychotherapy* 2008; **36**:675–83.

Additional resources

Further reading:

Department of Health. *Treatment Choice in Psychological Therapies and Counselling*. HMSO, 2001.

Devinsky O, Schachter S, Pacia S. *Complementary and Alternative Therapies for Epilepsy*. Demos, 2005.

Schacter SC, Schmidt D (eds). *Vagus Nerve Stimulation*, 2nd edn. Martin Dunitz, 2003.

Further reading on CBT:

- **The 'Overcoming' series**, published by Constable & Robinson (www.overcoming.co.uk; accessed August 2011). A large series of self-help books which use the theories and concepts of CBT to help people overcome many common problems. Titles include: overcoming social anxiety and shyness, overcoming depression and overcoming low self-esteem.

Useful CBT web links:

Royal College of Psychiatrists leaflet, www.rcpsych.ac.uk/mentalhealthinfoforall/treatments/cbt.aspx. This leaflet may be downloaded, printed out, photocopied and distributed free of charge as long as the Royal College of Psychiatrists is properly credited and no profit is gained from its use.

- **British Association for Behavioural and Cognitive Psychotherapies** website, www.babcp.com.
- **Calipso** website, www.calipso.co.uk.

(All accessed August 2011.)

Free online CBT resources:

- **Mood Gym**, moodgym.anu.edu.au. Information, quizzes, games and skills training to help prevent depression.
- **Living Life to the Full**, www.livinglifetothefull.com. Free, online life skills course for people feeling distressed, and their carers. Helps you understand why you feel as you do and make changes in your thinking, activities, sleep and relationships.
- **Fear Fighter**, www.fearfighter.com (free access can only be prescribed by your doctor in England and Wales).
- **Beating the Blues**, www.ultrasis.com/products/product.jsp?product_id = 1 (free access can only be prescribed by your doctor in England and Wales).

(All accessed August 2011.)

Further information on VNS:

- http://eu.cyberonics.com/en, Cyberonics home page (accessed August 2011).

Further information on ketogenic diet:

- **Great Ormond Street Hospital (GOSH)** www.gosh.nhs.uk (accessed August 2011); type 'ketogenic diet' into the website search box.
- **Matthew's Friends** www.matthewsfriends.org (accessed August 2011). Information and support for parents of children who are on the diet, or for parents who are thinking of starting their child on the diet.

Contacts for further information on non-drug treatments generally:

- **The epilepsy charities** – see Appendix.
- **Anxiety UK (formerly National Phobics Society)** Website www.anxietyuk.org.uk (accessed August 2011); email: info@anxietyuk.org.uk.
- **Depression Alliance** Helpline: 44 (0)845 123 23 20; email: information@depressionalliance.org.

CHAPTER 6

Prolonged or Repeated Seizures

Matthew C. Walker

UCL Institute of Neurology, University College London and National Hospital for Neurology and Neurosurgery, London, UK

OVERVIEW

- Continuous seizure activity for 30 minutes or longer (status epilepticus) is associated with neurological deficits, cognitive decline and a high mortality rate (10–20%)

- Management of prolonged seizures should be started as soon as possible by ensuring the patient is in a safe place with careful cardio-respiratory monitoring and treatment with either rectal diazepam or buccal midazolam

- Urgent admission to hospital is needed for further monitoring, investigations and more intensive treatment

- If someone is at danger of prolonged seizures or has had a history of serial seizures or status epilepticus, then there should be a plan in place for emergency management in the community

Single seizures are brief and usually without consequence. However, continuous seizure activity for 30 minutes or longer (status epilepticus) is associated with neurological deficits, cognitive decline and a high mortality rate (10–20%). People with epilepsy rarely go straight into status epilepticus; usually there is a premonitory phase of an increasing frequency of seizures. In order to prevent status epilepticus, early, expeditious treatment is required. Moreover, prolonged seizures often recur in those predisposed to such. Therefore if a prolonged seizure or a cluster of seizures has occurred in an individual then there should be a strategy in place to prevent subsequent episodes of status epilepticus.

Most seizures last less than 2 minutes (the post-ictal phase can last much longer: 10–20 minutes). Therefore, if seizures last for more than 5 minutes or are repeated without full recovery between, then immediate treatment is required. Such cases should be treated as an emergency. There is good evidence about how to manage status epilepticus, and those offering emergency treatment should be aware of local and national protocols.

ABC of Epilepsy, First Edition.
Edited by W. Henry Smithson and Matthew C. Walker.
© 2012 Blackwell Publishing Ltd. Published 2012 by Blackwell Publishing Ltd.

Treatment of prolonged or repeated generalised convulsive seizures

Treatment is more successful the earlier it is instigated, and therefore treatment should often be initiated before the patient reaches hospital. The aim is to terminate the seizure, with minimal respiratory or cardiac impairment while keeping the patient safe from accidental injury.

Ensure the patient is in a safe place. This has to be accomplished quickly while other treatment is being prepared. For instance, move the patient from a busy road, a water hazard or prevent the patient from falling downstairs. Assess the patient's cardiac and respiratory status and clear and maintain the airway. Medication should be rapidly administered and, in the premonitory phase, the choice lies between rectal diazepam, administered by trained personnel usually at a dose of 10–20 mg in adults (0.2–0.5 mg/kg in children) or midazolam given buccally (2.5–10 mg, depending on age). Midazolam is the preferred drug in many protocols (especially in children), and has recently been licensed for use in children.

If intravenous access is available, then lorazepam (2–4 mg in adults, 0.1 mg/kg in children) should be given.

Emergency admission by ambulance should be considered if seizures continue for more than five minutes after rescue medication, if there is a high risk of recurrence (if possible, see the patient's care plan), or that continued monitoring of the patient may be problematic, or if this is the first prolonged or repeated episode.

On admission to hospital, the following regimen is recommended.

The airway should be maintained, cardiac and respiratory function should be assessed, and high concentrations of oxygen should be given; gain intravenous access and check the finger-prick blood sugar. If hypoglycaemia is suspected then intravenous glucose with or without thiamine should be given. Blood should be sent for testing of electrolytes, calcium, glucose and full blood count.

Lorazepam intravenously, 2–4 mg should be given and repeated after 10 minutes if necessary (diazepam is an alternative, if lorazepam is not available). If a repeated dose of lorazepam is necessary, then the person should also be loaded with 15–20 mg/kg intravenous phenytoin with ECG monitoring at 50 mg/minute. If seizures continue then the person should be intubated and moved to an intensive therapy unit, where anaesthesia is instigated.

Treatment of non-convulsive status

In this condition, no convulsion is apparent. Diagnosis can be difficult because often, in non-convulsive status epilepticus, people are conscious and retain some awareness. It can therefore present with confusion, obtundation or even psychiatric symptoms. Cyclical symptoms may give a clue that this is due to an epileptic rather than psychiatric or other medical state. Diagnosis usually requires an EEG. Non-convulsive status epilepticus is probably underdiagnosed through failure to suspect the condition, especially in the elderly. It usually responds well to benzodiazepines. Whether emergency treatment with intravenous medication is required remains a matter of debate. Nevertheless, all people with this condition should be referred for specialist advice.

It is not unusual for people to have repeated episodes. Therefore if someone has had an episode of non-convulsive status epilepticus, then provision should be made for rapid treatment in the community – often an oral benzodiazepine such as clobazam is sufficient to terminate the event. Treatment resulting in the termination of the non-convulsive status epilepticus will often result in post-ictal confusion lasting minutes, meaning that clinical response to treatment may not be immediately obvious.

Prevention of status epilepticus

All people with epilepsy and their relative/carers should be given advice about prolonged seizures or repeat seizures/seizure clusters. If someone is at danger of prolonged seizures or has had a history of serial seizures or status epilepticus, then there should be a plan in place for emergency management in the community. For convulsions, this will be rectal diazepam, buccal midazolam or, in rare instances, rectal paraldehyde. For non-convulsive status epilepticus, this may be oral benzodiazepines (see above).

Further reading

http://www.epilepsysociety.org.uk/Forprofessionals/Articles-1   A link to the study guide for the International League against Epilepsy neurology specialist registrar's training weekend. See Chapters 33 and 34 by Professor M. Walker.

CHAPTER 7

Special Groups – Women, Children, Learning Disability and the Elderly

Jan Bagshaw[1], Colin D. Ferrie[2] and Mike P. Kerr[3]

[1]Community Epilepsy Services, Rochdale, UK
[2]Leeds General Infirmary, Leeds, UK
[3]Welsh Centre for Learning Disabilities, Cardiff, UK

OVERVIEW

- Certain groups of people with epilepsy present additional challenges.
- Children have a high incidence of epilepsy, and the seizure disorders can vary. A syndromic diagnosis is of particular importance as is the choice of correct AED.
- Women with epilepsy should be given guidance about contraception, conception, childbearing and hormonal change as well as the risks and benefits of taking AEDs during pregnancy.
- Some AEDs increase the rate of major congenital malformation, but women should be counselled not to stop taking their AEDs without seeking advice.
- People with learning disability are at a high risk of epilepsy and require expert management.
- Epilepsy is increasingly common in older people, and the resulting challenges are also discussed.

In this interestingly heterogeneous condition, the principles of care (a correct diagnosis, tailored treatment, structured monitoring, information provision and support, and a reassessment of the patient if seizure type or frequency changes) should be accessible to all patients. In some groups, having epilepsy produces additional challenges. This chapter considers four such groups: children, women, people with learning disability and the elderly.

Children

Epilepsy is more common in children than in any other age group apart from the geriatric population. Indeed epileptic seizures are more likely to occur on the first day of life than at any other time. The rate of new-onset seizures and epilepsy thereafter falls steeply but remains high throughout infancy, dropping further during childhood and into adolescence.

Although idiopathic epilepsies occur throughout childhood, seizures occurring in babies and infants often have an underlying cause. This can have important genetic and management implications. For example, pyridoxine-dependent seizures are autosomal recessive disorders which do not respond to conventional antiepileptic drugs but do respond to pyridoxine. Moreover, epilepsies in this age group, more than at any other age, can be associated with developmental problems, which may be partially preventable by early seizure control. For these reasons, seizure disorders presenting in this age group should generally be referred promptly to a paediatric neurologist.

Early, mid to late childhood is characterised by the occurrence of many well-defined epilepsy syndromes. Correct diagnosis of these is important for optimal management and accurate prognostication. Many of these syndromes are idiopathic, often with excellent prognoses. Managing them can be very rewarding to the clinician. Unfortunately a number of severe epilepsies also occur in this age group. These can occur in children who have hitherto been developing normally, and can be accompanied by severe cognitive and behavioural problems. Early identification of these can curtail unnecessary investigations and can help the family begin the inevitably difficult adjustments required. Children in this age group are usually managed by paediatricians with special expertise in epilepsy. However, there should be a well-defined, accessible local network to ensure that further expertise, usually from a paediatric neurologist, can be obtained if diagnosis or management is proving problematic. It is recommended that children who continue to have seizures after two antiepileptic drugs have been tried should be reviewed by a paediatric neurologist.

Inevitably young children are relatively passive recipients of care. Usually their parents act as advocates for them. Once children can effectively communicate they should be actively involved in their care. If a history is not obtained from them, important diagnostic information will be lost. Their perceptions of the impact of their epilepsy should be sought. Most children require time and encouragement to tell professionals how they really feel. Provision of relevant information to children is important, and many older children are active surfers of the internet.

Knowledge about epilepsy among teaching staff is often poor. The clinical team responsible for a child with epilepsy should ensure that the school has appropriate knowledge of the condition. Each child should have an individual care plan specifying how each reasonably foreseeable problem should be dealt with. Training on the use of rescue mediation may need to be arranged. Advice

ABC of Epilepsy, First Edition.
Edited by W. Henry Smithson and Matthew C. Walker.
© 2012 Blackwell Publishing Ltd. Published 2012 by Blackwell Publishing Ltd.

on safety matters, seeking to maximise the child's participation in all school activities, is likely to be needed.

Older children and adolescents should begin to take responsibility for their drug treatment. They, as well as their parents, should be asked how AEDs make them feel. Adherence to medication is likely to be improved if they have been involved in decision-making. The teenage period is often characterised by rebellion and pushing at boundaries. This time can be particularly tough for those with epilepsy. As well as all the other issues, real and imaginary, faced by teenagers, those with epilepsy may have to cope with additional restrictions on their freedom, and the realisation that certain activities, such as driving, and certain fields of employment, may not be open to them. Self-image may be distorted and self-esteem low. Parents, teachers and even health professionals may be unduly pessimistic about the future.

Transition to adult services is often feared by parents. Some teenagers with epilepsy share this concern; others probably look forward to it. There are different models of achieving transition to adult services. What is important is that the patient and their families feel supported through it and know who to contact if difficulties arise. The handover offers an opportunity for fresh eyes to look at the young person with epilepsy.

Women

Fertility, preconceptual counselling and pregnancy

Women with treated epilepsy have lower fertility rates than an age-matched general population, and the causes may be complex and result in part from social and relationship effects of epilepsy, and from personal choice not to have children because of concerns about 'passing on the condition', as well as genetic factors and AED effects.

Nevertheless, counselling should be offered to all women of child-bearing age as soon after diagnosis as possible and continue at follow up visits, whether or not pregnancy is actively planned. Paediatric and adolescence handover clinics should offer appropriate information and support. Currently there seems to be a shortfall in such information provision, with a survey showing that only 38–48% of women recalled being given information on contraception, post-coital contraception, folic acid and teratogenicity (Bell *et al.*, 2002). The risks and benefits of reducing or changing medication should be discussed and accurately documented. It is equally important to discuss the risk of fetal malformations. A register of pregnancies in women with epilepsy (The UK and Ireland Epilepsy and Pregnancy Register; Box 7.1) has been collecting data about major congenital malformations (MCMs) for over 10 years, and now has about 8000 registrations. This register shows that the vast majority of women with epilepsy have a normal pregnancy, with an overall rate of MCMs of about 4.2%. The MCM rate for women with epilepsy who had not taken AEDs is 2.2%; so, while women should take early advice about their pregnancy, they should not stop their medication before advice because of the risk of seizures. The MCM rate for polytherapy exposure is greater than for monotherapy exposure. Polytherapy regimens containing valproate have significantly more MCMs than those not containing valproate. For monotherapy exposures, carbamazepine is associated with the lowest risk of MCM.

Box 7.1 UK and Ireland epilepsy and pregnancy register

Data from the register show that the incidence of major congenital malformations is as follows:

- All monotherapy 3.4%:
  - carbamazepine 2.4%
  - all valproate 6.3%:
    low-dose valproate, <1000 mg/day 5%
    high-dose valproate, >1000 mg/day 9.1%
  - lamotrigine 2.7%:
    doses <400 mg/day 2.4%
    doses >400 mg/day 5.9%
- Polytherapy 6.0%:
  - polytherapy not containing valproate 4.2%
  - polytherapy containing valproate 8.9%
- No AED 2.2% (just above background incidence).

The prescription of 5 mg of folic acid daily, before conception and at least until the end of the first trimester, is recommended on an empirical basis in women with epilepsy. This can reduce the risk of recurrent neural tube defect, but as yet there is little evidence that folic acid will safeguard against the neural tube defects seen in association with AEDs. There have been some concerns that folic acid may exacerbate seizures, but these fears have generally been unsupported. In addition, women on an enzyme-inducing drug (e.g. carbamazepine) should be recommended to take vitamin K in the last month of pregnancy.

A more recent concern is that children exposed to antiepileptic drugs in utero may perform less well at school, with a higher rate of statements of special educational needs. This risk is apparent with valproate but not carbamazepine (studies of other AEDs have not had the power to determine safety or otherwise). In one study, five or more tonic–clonic seizures during pregnancy also had an effect on the fetus – approximately equivalent to valproate. Stopping medication before or during pregnancy may also expose the woman to the risk of status epilepticus or sudden unexpected death in epilepsy. Overall, women should be on the least amount of medication that adequately controls their epilepsy and preferably not on regimens containing valproate.

During pregnancy, the pharmacokinetics of AEDs can change dramatically, and careful monitoring of seizures and AED levels is required, especially in the last trimester.

Because of the increased risk of complications during pregnancy and the potential teratogenic effect of taking AEDs, women with epilepsy need to be encouraged to plan their pregnancies, whether they are presently experiencing seizures or not. This guidance should be provided by an experienced professional with expert knowledge of epilepsy, working in partnership with women, supporting informed decisions regarding the most appropriate treatment. Together the aim is to achieve a good seizure control, taking medication that carries the lowest teratogenic risk; at the same time acknowledging that for some women, good seizure control can only be achieved on their usual dose of AED therapy.

The benefits of breast feeding probably outweigh the exposure of the baby to low levels of AEDs contained in breast milk; the possible exception being phenobarbital. Babies being breast fed by women on polytherapy or on drugs that are expressed at reasonable concentrations in breast milk should be watched for signs of irritability, feeding problems or excessive drowsiness.

Contraception and antiepileptic drugs

It is of paramount importance that women with epilepsy access accurate/current advice and information regarding contraception and AEDs. AEDs do not lower the effectiveness of depot medroxyprogesterone acetate (Depo-Provera), intrauterine devices and intrauterine systems. While oestrogen is potentially proconvulsant, the oral contraceptive pill as a rule has no undesirable effects on the epilepsy. Cautious consideration should be given when prescribing the oral contraceptive pill in clients with difficult epilepsy and those with a history of status epilepticus. Enzyme-inducing AEDs (Table 7.1) increase the rate at which the steroid content of the pill is metabolised. These drugs consequently have the potential to decrease the efficacy of low-oestrogen contraceptives containing less than 50 μg of oestrogenic hormone. There is no risk with non-enzyme-inducing drugs. Despite the risk, inappropriate prescribing of low-oestrogen contraceptives with enzyme-inducing drugs is widespread (Kitson, 2000).

The menopause

Increases in seizure frequency are not uncommon around the menopause. However, menopause itself is not consistently associated with any particular change in seizure frequency; nevertheless, the pattern of seizures may change and become less predictable. Moreover, some people find that their seizure frequency can change after menopause (some have an increase, some a decrease).

There are no consistent data on the effect of hormone replacement therapy on seizure frequency – again both decreases and increases in seizure frequency can occur. In the same way that antiepileptic drugs interact with the oral contraceptive pill, so they can interact with hormone replacement therapy.

Because of the effects of antiepileptic drugs on bone density, menopausal woman on antiepileptic drug therapy should have their bone density monitored.

Table 7.1 Contraception and antiepileptic drugs.

AED	Effect on oral contraceptive pill	Effect on AED
Carbamazepine Oxcarbazepine Topiramate Phenytoin Phenobarbital	Enzyme inducers that reduce the effectiveness of oestrogen: a minimum of 50 μg oestrogen preparation is required	Oestrogen may have a proconvulsant effect
Felbamate Valproate	Nil or may increase hormone levels	
Lamotrigine Gabapentin Levetiracetam Tiagabine	No effect on hormonal levels	Oral contraceptive pill reduces serum level of lamotrigine

People with a learning disability

When delivering epilepsy care to people with a learning disability, certain reasonable adjustments are needed by the clinician so that management meets the often more complex requirements of these individuals. These requirements relate to the overlap of co-morbidities in this population, in particular physical, neurological and psychiatric. Adjusting for the physical co-morbidities includes recognition that concurrent unrecognised medical conditions are more frequent, such as reflux oesophagitis, and may explain appetite or behavioural change. A further physical issue is the presence of dysphagia and potential that an individual may need percutaneous endoscopic gastrostomy (PEG) feeding and adjustment in the mode of AED delivery.

Neurological disabilities are related to the complexity and syndromic nature of the epilepsy that has been addressed elsewhere in this book.

It is however the psychological issues that most influence the epilepsy and its management.

Epilepsy is associated with high rates of emotional and behavioural disturbance. In people with a learning disability the key impact appears to be that of seizures on mental well being. Direct seizure impact such as post-ictal psychosis is rare, though it should still be part of any clinical enquiry.

Concurrent behavioural disturbance or associated autistic features are common and this can cause confusion over diagnosis and can make investigation and haematological monitoring difficult. Co-prescription of antipsychotic medication can influence seizure frequency.

Lastly, as we have already discussed, behavioural change during treatment needs careful assessment for attribution.

These common associations with psychological ill health can lead to specialist care being provided by psychiatric rather than neurological services, and referral pathways should reflect this.

Older people

Epilepsy in the older person is potentially more serious than in the younger population. An older person may worry, not without reason, that future seizures may lead to injury. The risk of injury from falls during a seizure is increased due to frailty, including osteoporotic fractures. This can mark a watershed in the person's life, after which there can be a remarkable decline in functional independence. This in turn may lead to a loss of confidence. A fear of further falls can severely limit both physical activity and social contact, sometimes rendering the person housebound and resulting in them becoming dependant on others. Where there are prolonged post-ictal states (more common in older people), this obviously adds to the potential hazards.

Fear of an adverse reaction to the diagnosis from both family and friends, and exclusion from some activities (e.g. less involvement with grandchildren, loss of driving licence) can lead to isolation, depression, felt or enacted stigma, and feelings of impending doom. This all contributes to the process of disempowerment.

Managing epilepsy in older people is more than just drug treatment. The problem of epilepsy for the person, and the impact of seizures, goes far beyond their immediate consequences (Baker *et al.*, 2001). Many older people may have childhood memories that go back to a time when epilepsy was stigmatised and seizures were, in general, poorly controlled. They may hold many misconceptions and myths about epilepsy. A positive approach is paramount in giving reassurance that, in the vast majority of cases, seizures do not indicate serious brain damage, that epilepsy itself rarely causes further damage to the brain, and that the condition is unrelated to any psychiatric disturbance (not forgetting to emphasise that both can be controlled by medication).

Education, information and support are of equal importance. The advice in this age group is the same as that given to any people with epilepsy. An opportunity to air their beliefs, preconceptions and worries is essential. This will not be achieved in a single consultation. Follow-up appointments are crucial. A review of an individual's circumstances to optimise their mobility arrangements and domestic situation should be undertaken and a referral made to the multidisciplinary team as appropriate. The tendency of carers, supporters and relatives to discourage patients from living a full and independent life should be anticipated.

Acute symptomatic seizures are most suitably managed by treating the underlying precipitant. AED therapy may be necessary in some circumstances, on a temporary basis, to suppress seizures while control of the underlying illness is achieved.

There is an enormous amount of literature on AED therapy. However, it contains little specific reference to older people. Even in those few drug trials from which older people are not actually excluded, they are seriously underrepresented. Information regarding seizure recurrence after a first seizure, and the response to treatment, is scant. Such data are necessary to weigh the risks of epilepsy and its complications against drug treatment and the associated side effects. Polypharmacy is common in older people, therefore increasing the risk of AED interactions and adverse effects. AEDs may cause acute dose-related or idiosyncratic side effects. This may present subtly in an older person, who may have pre-existing pathology impairing either cognitive function or mobility. Age-related pharmacokinetic changes require a reduced daily dose of AEDs, but decisions about treatment are pragmatic. Patients with recurrent unprovoked seizures clearly require treatment. Although a range of antiepileptic drugs can be used as initial treatment in older people, the evidence supports the preferential use of lamotirigine, gabapentin, topiratmate (at low dose), valproate (cautiously due to tremor and sedation) and levetiracetam.

Whichever drug is used, the introductory dose should be low and dose titration should be slow and cautious to avoid adverse effects. Monitoring for potential side effects should be intensive and due consideration should be given to the presentation of non-specific side effects of AEDs. Ideally treatment should be with monotherapy. Therapeutic ranges are less helpful in the older population.

AED pharmacokinetics may be altered by age. It should be emphasised that inter-individual variability may be much more important than changes associated with age alone. Tailoring of the dose with regard to co-morbidity and other medication is paramount to avoid toxicity.

References

Arain AM, Abou-Khalil BW. Management of new-onset epilepsy in the elderly. *Nat. Rev. Neurol.* 2009; **5**(7):363–71.

Baker GA, Jacoby A, Buck D, Brooks J, Potts P, Chadwick DW. The quality of life of older people with epilepsy: findings from a UK community study. *Seizure* 2001; **10**(2):92–9.

Bell GS, Nashef L, Kendall S, Solomon J, Poole K, Johnson AL *et al.* Information recalled by women taking anti-epileptic drugs for epilepsy: a questionnaire study. *Epilepsy Research* 2002; **52**(2):139–46.

Kitson A. Services for Patients with Epilepsy: Report of a CSAG Committee Chaired by Professor Alison Kitson. Department of Health, 2000.

Further reading

Appleton R, Chappell B, Berne M. *Epilepsy and Your Child*, 2nd edn. Class Publishing, 2004.

Betts T. *Epilepsy in Women (the Facts)*. Oxford University Press, 2008.

Kutscher ML. *Children with Seizures: A Guide for Parents, Teachers and Other Professionals*. Jessica Kingsley Publishers, 2006.

Morrow J. *The XX Factor: Treating Women with Anti-Epileptic Drugs*. National Services for Health Improvement, 2007.

Prasher VP, Kerr M. *Epilepsy and Intellectual Disabilities*. Springer, 2008.

CHAPTER 8

Monitoring and Review – How to Manage the Condition Long Term

Colin D. Ferrie[1], Alice Hanscomb[2] and Mike P. Kerr[3]

[1]Leeds General Infirmary, Leeds, UK
[2]Hanscomb Training & Consultancy, High Wycombe, UK
[3]Welsh Centre for Learning Disabilities, Cardiff, UK

OVERVIEW

- A review of epilepsy should include a review of the diagnosis, effect and side effects of treatment, lifestyle advice and social and psychological factors, provision of information and whether referral is needed
- Good communication between the clinician and those involved with the condition – the individual and sometimes their family or carers – is central to an effective review
- Epilepsy is not just about having symptoms of seizures – it is far more complex, and the social and psychological issues must be considered
- Children with epilepsy should be reviewed regularly by the clinician principally responsible for their care
- Reasonable adjustments are needed by the clinician so that management of people with learning disability meets the often more complex requirements of these individuals
- The role of the specialist nurse in supporting not only the patient but also healthcare professionals is invaluable
- This chapter includes some reflections from patients, which have been told to the authors over the years

'Healthcare professionals should adopt a consulting style that enables the individual with epilepsy to participate as a partner in all decisions about healthcare.'

– NICE guideline CG20

The annual review is a key part in managing the epilepsies; both for the person with the condition and the clinician. It gives the medical professional a chance to hear the whole picture of the person's situation and to ask key questions in order to tailor the treatment appropriately to the person's current needs. People with epilepsy value the time during the review to ask questions and inform the clinician as to how effective the treatment is, and to discuss treatment options and lifestyle issues.

'The annual review was an opportunity to be given information to enable me to make informed decisions about my condition and also to tell a professional how having epilepsy and seizures affected me.'

Regular review creates a partnership, and it is the teamwork that comes out of that partnership that stands the best chance of optimising not only seizure control but also individual quality of life. Good communication between the clinician and those involved with the condition – the individual and sometimes their family or carers – is therefore central to an effective review.

'The doctor's words stay with the person all day, all month, all year. I look forward to seeing you for a long time.'

Without information neither party can play their part in the effective management of the condition. Without sound communication, rapport and trust, any information gained by either party can be rendered sterile. People need to be actively encouraged to ask questions and be really involved in the process. Some people may feel anxious and disempowered during the consultation, so the clinician needs to take this into account and consult in such a way as to reduce this as effectively as possible.

Communication is at the heart of what people with epilepsy want from their annual reviews, which is:

- for the clinician to have read previous review notes;
- honest two-way communication that fosters mutual trust and respect;
- to have their condition reviewed in the light of their particular situation;
- to have a comprehensive discussion to assess their epilepsy, the treatment and how either is affecting their current quality of life;
- to be central in the discussion about their condition. For those who find communication difficult it is important to involve a carer who really knows them and to have a three-way conversation;
- with children, to involve them as well as the parents as much as possible;
- to be encouraged to ask questions and given time to have them answered;

ABC of Epilepsy, First Edition.
Edited by W. Henry Smithson and Matthew C. Walker.
© 2012 Blackwell Publishing Ltd. Published 2012 by Blackwell Publishing Ltd.

- to be given objective information on the risks of epilepsy, the implications of not taking AEDs and how to minimise those risks. Discussion about the risk of SUDEP is of particular importance;
- to be given clear information on which to base decisions on treatments, life choices, such as family planning, school issues, driving etc.;
- to have the epilepsy assessed in the context of their quality of life, not just their seizures;
- encouragement to make notes, acknowledging that it can be a lot to remember;
- to have their family and carers appropriately involved;
- for the language used to be patient friendly and age appropriate;
- to be given details of further sources of information and support: specialist nurses, charity resources such as websites, self-help and helplines (information about national and specialist epilepsy charities is available in the Appendix);
- to have any concerns taken seriously and acknowledged, even if there is little, if anything, a clinician can do about them; acknowledgement of concerns is important to the relationship;
- to have access to specialist help by phone/email between reviews;
- to be offered referral to tertiary centres if needs be.

People with epilepsy also find it valuable to have contact with clinicians between reviews. This can be accomplished by phone or email. The impact of worsening side effects or increased seizures on quality of life can be enormous, especially if the GP has limited knowledge of the condition and is unable to make changes.

Having access to specialist advice in these situations can be vital when an individual's epilepsy is resistant to treatment and may deteriorate suddenly with potentially life-threatening consequences. It is crucial that the clinician does not just 'seizure count'; especially when improvement in seizure control is gained at the expense of side effects. There may be times in a person's life when the seizures are more acceptable to them than the side effects; being clear which is most important to the person with the condition at the time is, therefore, critical. And, of course the previous review needs to be read in advance of seeing the person the next time: nothing is more disheartening than running out of time in a review because the clinician asks lots of questions that were covered in the last review, simply because the notes from the previous meeting haven't been adequately made or had not been read.

The clinical requirements of the review depend on the type of epilepsy, associated co-morbidity, and frequency and nature of seizures. Epilepsy review can be offered in both primary and secondary care and also in 'intermediate clinics' run by either specialist nurses or general practitioners with a special interest.

People with learning disability

People with complex health needs will require input from a variety of professionals in a number of different settings. Ensuring good communication both between individual and professional and between different professionals is crucial to optimal care. Time should be set aside to ensure a relaxed consultation to allow for a clear understanding of the implications of epilepsy and the treatment. Systems should be in place to ensure good and timely communication between professionals and to define the responsibilities of each member of the team.

> 'Always clarify that the person understands – they are on sedating anticonvulsants – they may say they get what you are saying but may not!'

Children

Most children with epilepsy are managed principally within secondary care by paediatricians. Children with significant co-morbidities, such as cerebral palsy, learning difficulties and severe behavioural problems are usually cared for by community paediatricians and consultants in neurodisability. Children with more severe epilepsy are usually managed by tertiary-level paediatric neurologists, often jointly with secondary-based paediatricians/ community paediatricians and neurodisability consultants. All children with epilepsy should have access to an epilepsy nurse. Unfortunately such services remain patchy. Primary care generally has a limited role, mainly involving repeat prescribing of AEDs and being the first point of contact when problems arise. Ensuring parents understand this complex system is important if children with epilepsy are to receive optimal care.

Children with epilepsy should be reviewed regularly by the clinician principally responsible for their care. This should be at least yearly, but more frequently in most. In addition to assessing seizure frequency and AED monitoring, there should be a focus on assessing co-morbidities which are common in children with epilepsy. Most clinicians who care for children with epilepsy have only limited training in managing these, and there should be clear local referral pathways to enable children with epilepsy to access appropriate services.

> 'Always remember or try to remember how hard it is in the outside world for the person – the prejudice that exists the moment the person says they have the condition and even more so when they have a seizure in front of someone – don't be dismissive.'

It is generally considered that children with epilepsy that has not been controlled with two antiepileptic drugs should be referred to a paediatric neurologist. An important reason for this is to review whether the child should be considered for surgical treatment for their epilepsy or for non-drug treatments such as the ketogenic diet.

Children spend a considerable proportion of their awake time at school, and school issues often loom large. At review the clinician should assess if there are epilepsy-related issues at school which need to be addressed. School liaison is usually an important role of the paediatric epilepsy nurse.

Key principles of review

While the functions of each setting are distinct, there are some key principles underpinning epilepsy review.

- Review the diagnosis to ensure the correct classification and aetiology.
- Review the treatment: some epilepsy syndromes require specific treatment.
- Check the nature and frequency of seizures but remember self-report is unreliable.
- Discuss medicines adherence.
- Discuss lifestyle changes as appropriate.
- Provide and record information needs.
- Consider onward referral in certain circumstances (e.g. change in seizure frequency or pattern, pregnancy, uncertain diagnosis, treatment side effects, refractory seizures).
- Agree date and form of the next review.

> 'I remember when I was told I was at risk of SUDEP or having a fatal accident during a seizure. I appreciated the consultant being straight with me. Information generally empowered me and made me reflect on my self- management skills.'

The role of primary care

The majority of people with epilepsy can expect good seizure control, and monitoring by specialist services is not necessary. The benefit of regular review has been reinforced by epilepsy being part of the general practice clinical quality and outcome framework. A member of the practice team should be identified as having particular responsibility for epilepsy care. In smaller practices this may be difficult, and in a federated structure of co-operation between practices, it may be decided to have practitioners with a special interest who could review all stable patients with epilepsy in a group of practices.

The role of secondary care

The more specialised expertise should be focused on people with refractory epilepsy, where there is diagnostic doubt or when epilepsy is part of a more complex clinical picture. This is particularly so in people with learning disability, in older people and when women with epilepsy are considering pregnancy.

> 'When seeing a registrar – which is often the case – it would be useful for them to have read the case history before, as often they seem like they don't know anything about me but pretend they have.'

The role of intermediate care

The specialist team should include a neurologist and an epilepsy specialist nurse (ESN), the pivotal team member, who will help to ensure a seamless service between primary and secondary care and all relevant healthcare professionals. Having a dedicated specialist team helps to ensure continuity of care and development of good relationships with patients.

> 'Epilepsy is not just about having symptoms of seizures – it is far more complex. Sometimes I have been more disabled by the social and psychological issues than the physical symptoms of seizures.'

The role of the ESN in supporting not only the patient but also healthcare professionals is invaluable, providing medication monitoring, education, counselling and as a resource of information.

It is of paramount importance that the service is easy to access. Referrals will be received from healthcare professionals. Self-referrals from patients with a confirmed diagnosis will help to reduce the length of time of accessing the service. A telephone helpline can allow timely expert advice and emergency intervention to reduce appointments with general practitioners, contact with Accident and Emergency services and hospital admissions.

An intermediate clinic will call on the expertise of neurologists, epilepsy nurse specialists, and in some areas also general practitioners with a special interest. Generally the nurse specialist provides a link between services. A clinic in Rochdale, for instance, provides appointments for epilepsy patients with an established diagnosis who are seen within a community clinic; home visits that are arranged as appropriate, with the location and time negotiated to suit patient and service needs; education and training in all aspects of epilepsy to healthcare professionals and care staff; road shows/exhibitions to the general public on request; and a resource facility for primary, secondary and social care staff and to the general public.

Further reading

Patsalos PN, Berry DJ, Bourgeois BF, Cloyd JC, Glauser TA, Johannessen SI *et al.* Antiepileptic drugs – best practice guidelines for therapeutic drug monitoring: a position paper by the subcommission on therapeutic drug monitoring, ILAE Commission on Therapeutic Strategies. *Epilepsia* 2008; **49**(7):1239–76.

Stokes T, Shaw EJ, Juarez-Garcia A, Camosso-Stefinovic J, Baker R. Appendix A: Differential diagnosis of epilepsy, in *Clinical Guidelines and Evidence Review for the Epilepsies: Diagnosis and Management in Adults and Children in Primary and Secondary Care* (NICE Clinical Guideline CG20). Royal College of General Practitioners, 2004.

CHAPTER 9

Living with Epilepsy – Information, Support and Self-Management

Alice Hanscomb[1] and W. Henry Smithson[2]

[1]Hanscomb Training & Consultancy, High Wycombe, UK
[2]Academic Unit of Primary Medical Care, Medical School, University of Sheffield, Sheffield, UK

OVERVIEW

- All individuals with a long-term condition make sense of this in their own way and take individual decisions about how best to manage themselves and their condition
- Living with epilepsy can have detrimental impact on the individual. Having knowledge and information can lessen this impact. The needs of the individual and the resources available are listed below
- Epilepsy is not without risks. SUDEP is more common in people with generalised unwitnessed nocturnal seizures, remote symptomatic epilepsy, neuropathological abnormality, learning disability, poor AED adherence, concurrent psychotropic medication, in the young, males, and with alcohol abuse or abrupt dose change, but the risk can be reduced by good seizure control

---

Living with epilepsy can be immensely difficult. It is far from being 'just' a medical condition, and can have debilitating psychological and social ramifications. This burden is not just about having seizures and taking potentially toxic medications, but about the fear of having a seizure, either alone where there could be risk of injury or even SUDEP (see page 31), or in public in front of others (just dropping a cup of coffee in a restaurant or tripping on a pavement can cause most of us great embarrassment). A counsellor who has epilepsy described having the condition as 'walking on a series of trap doors, not knowing when one might open and throw you to the ground'. The diagnosis of epilepsy may result in the loss of self-esteem, independence, job and income, and the reality of losing your driving licence and loss of control over one's life. This 'loss response' of initial shock, anger and even denial, together with guilt or blame (in some ways similar to bereavement) has to be worked through before the individual can accept and manage their lives with epilepsy. The clinician must support the individual through this loss response which may not be a 'one off' event but unpredictable and recurrent (see Box 9.1).

This statement, made by someone who has the condition, speaks volumes. It reminds clinicians to look at the person as a whole.

"Epilepsy is not just about having symptoms of seizures – it's far more complex. Sometimes I have been more disabled by the social and psychological issues than the physical symptoms of seizures."

Box 9.1 **The impact of epilepsy**

Key pieces of information may include:

- What epilepsy is, and the type of epilepsy they have
- Seizures being symptoms of a cerebral event
- Tests and what they involve, and what the tests may reveal or not reveal and why
- Possible cause for their condition and, if possible, prognosis
- Treatment options, including VNS, surgery and choices of medication
- How medication works and why it needs to be taken consistently
- What to do if there are side effects and what to expect
- Possible interactions with other medications
- Minimising risk of accidents and SUDEP
- Relevant life issues such as:
  - family planning
  - up-to-date driving regulations
  - school/work issues
  - travel and leisure issues
- Other sources of support, including epilepsy specialist nurses, councillors, psychologists etc.
- Charity contact details (see Box 9.2).

Box 9.2 **Charities**

Charities include:

- Epilepsy Action: helpline 0808 800 5050; www.epilepsy.org.uk
- Epilepsy Scotland: helpline 0800 800 2200; www.epilepsyscotland.org.uk
- Epilepsy Society: helpline 01494 601400; www.epilepsysociety.org.uk
- Joint Epilepsy Council: http://www.jointepilepsycouncil.org.uk/ for lists of other epilepsy charities

---

ABC of Epilepsy, First Edition.
Edited by W. Henry Smithson and Matthew C. Walker.
© 2012 Blackwell Publishing Ltd. Published 2012 by Blackwell Publishing Ltd.

Getting training in the psycho-social aspects of epilepsy is important. In training sessions for medical professionals, the (non-medical) trainer invites participants to ask themselves what it would be like to have epilepsy: which areas of their lives would be affected, how they would feel, what questions would they ask and where would they go for an answer. By doing this, the trainer sheds real light on what people have to do to live with the condition, and reinforces how the clinical world of diagnosis, seizure counting and classifying, and the identification of possible causes, syndromes and treatments is often a world apart from the patient.

Self-management

All individuals with a long-term condition make sense of this in their own way and take individual decisions about how best to manage themselves and their condition. This is of particular importance in epilepsy, where there is a feeling of loss of control. Self-management (comprising assimilation of medical management, living with the condition and the emotional response to this) leads to a management paradigm that can sit uncomfortably with some clinicians but offers an opportunity for patient and professional to work together towards 'shared decision-making' to optimise the decisions taken by the individual. This can result in the individual behaving in a way that takes control of the condition (self-efficacy).

People with epilepsy make decisions about medicines, lifestyle, seizure control, staying safe and using information. It is recognised that one of the reasons people do not become seizure free is because they are not taking the medication as prescribed. Some choose not to inform their clinician of any inconsistencies in their taking of AEDs. It may be that they do not think the clinician will understand why they are not taking the AEDs or won't want to know about their concerns, or may feel fearful of the clinician's reaction. Central to the concordant approach is identifying the persons own goals for managing their condition, and aligning the medical goals to suit the individual.

A discussion about how the patient takes their medicines, about their concerns around medication and epilepsy and a discussion of risks involved with non-adherence (seizure recurrence, accidents, and in a small number of people with particular seizures, even death) should be part of an annual review.

Support

Many people with epilepsy at some time experience anxiety and depression, particularly soon after diagnosis. This is often as a result of the psychological and social impact of the condition. As a result, it is important that psychological support is offered at diagnosis and beyond, and reassurance is given that it is perfectly normal and

understandable for people to experience worry and stress at having epilepsy with all its possible implications.

Some people with epilepsy benefit greatly from using epilepsy helplines to talk about their issues, fears and anxieties (see Box 9.3). Others may need formal counselling or other psychological help (see Chapter 5) that should be offered tactfully and with the understanding that these sources of help can be of benefit to anyone who has this condition because of the very real effects it can have on anyone, physically, psychologically and socially.

Box 9.3 **Helplines**

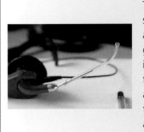

The charity helplines offer invaluable support and information. Some, such as the Epilepsy Society, specialise in giving emotional support as well as information, offering a caller-led confidential services which allows callers anonymity and the time they need to talk through all their issues, feelings and concerns.

Source: Photograph supplied with kind permission of Lukasz Abramowicz.

Epilepsy specialist nurses can provide excellent back up in providing information and support, and can give the person extra time to talk about their epilepsy in the context of their life issues.

Epilepsy is still dogged by stigma. This is partly due to the fact that it is one of the oldest known conditions and so has had many centuries to accumulate myths and misunderstandings. It is also because people know little about the condition and, of course, witnessing a seizure can be a terrifying experience. It is also unpredictable and 'hidden'. Stigma can be externally driven through colleagues, potential employers, teachers, health professionals, or even relatives and friends, or internally through 'self-stigmatisation', with low self-esteem and self-condemnation. This can be exacerbated if the knowledge the person has about the condition is particularly outdated, as may be the case in the older generations, as when they were growing up epilepsy may have been stigmatised to the extent that people with the condition where shut away in institutions and almost forgotten about by their relatives. So in the event of an older person being diagnosed, the unstated assumption may be that this will happen to them.

Also some cultures may have a particular view of the condition, so culturally applied stigma can cause specific distress; such as in cultures where epilepsy can be a block to marriage.

Sudden unexplained death in epilepsy

Epilepsy carries an excess mortality rate with a two- or threefold increase in standardised mortality over the general population. The causes of death are listed in Box 9.4.

SUDEP is defined in the UK as 'a sudden and unexpected witnessed or unwitnessed non-traumatic and non-drowning death in epilepsy with or without evidence for a seizure and excluding

Box 9.4 **Causes of death**

- Deaths unrelated to epilepsy
- Deaths from associated/underlying conditions
- Epilepsy related
- Seizure related
  - Status epilepticus
  - Drowning, burns, accidents related to seizures
  - The majority of sudden unexpected deaths
  - Deaths in a seizure due to asphyxiation
- Deaths due to medical or surgical treatment of epilepsy
- Suicide

Source: From Nashef and Langan (2004).

documented status epilepticus, where post mortem examination does not reveal a cause of death'. This definition does not presuppose a mechanism of death and it is likely that SUDEP may result from a variety of mechanisms resulting from the post-ictal features of hypoxia, autonomic disturbance, cardiac arrhythmia, pulmonary oedema and/or obstructive apnoea.

Until recently, the risk of death in epilepsy was not widely known, but with the work of epilepsy charities, both in the UK and abroad, it is now recognised as a risk to be managed.

The incidence of SUDEP ranges from 1/250 cases per year in refractory epilepsy in a co-morbid population to 1/2500 per year in people with infrequent seizures. In those with the most refractory epilepsy undergoing pre-surgical assessment, the risk is 1% per year. The UK national sentinel audit of epilepsy-related death proposed an incidence of about 1000 deaths a year in the UK, with over half due to SUDEP, and with a tragically high incidence in young adults (Hannah *et al.*, 2002). It is known that SUDEP is more common in people with generalised unwitnessed nocturnal seizures, remote symptomatic epilepsy, neuropathological abnormality, learning disability, poor AED adherence, concurrent psychotropic medication, in the young, males, and with alcohol abuse or abrupt dose change (Forsgren *et al.*, 2005), and it is also known that the risk of death reduces with better seizure control.

Advice to individuals and families about reducing the risk is available on a dedicated charity web page, www.sudep.org.

Providing information

It is important to have an understanding of the persons' life as well as their epilepsy before giving information. It is easy to fall into 'the information trap' and give information for information's sake, or to meet our own needs to be helpful, rather than tailoring the information to the needs of the person. This also has to be balanced against the considerable amount of often-inaccurate information available on the internet. There is so much information that a person needs at different stages of this condition, from diagnosis, going into puberty or menopause or starting school or starting a family. The information that is given needs to be appropriate to the person's needs at the time. So we need to provide accurate, tailored and appropriate information in the right way at the right time. The risk of SUDEP is

often an important discussion to allay fears in those whose seizures are well controlled, and to emphasise the importance of adherence and the dangers of sudden withdrawal or under-treatment.

People may remember only a small amount of information at any one time, particularly when anxious or stressed, so providing back-up information sources is important. It is difficult for the clinician to provide all necessary information in a time-limited service setting, but it is crucial that individuals are signposted to some excellent sources of help and support.

It is also important for the family to receive information and to be able to ask questions. It may also be relevant for the person's work place, school or care home to receive information about the condition too. Epilepsy will affect everyone connected with the person with the condition, and having good information and support for everyone concerned can make the difference between a breakdown of normal functioning or effective coping and managing.

It is often found that in the case of the very young, if the parents are coping well with their child's epilepsy, the child will most likely be able to do the same. Support of parents is therefore vital for a child's wellbeing.

In some instances, it may be important to provide information before it may actually be needed. An example of this would be when talking with a girl who is not yet of childbearing age: it may not yet be necessary to start talking about having children, but it could be very useful to inform the child (and possibly the parents) that there are issues on AEDs around contraception and its effectiveness which will need to be addressed when she becomes sexually active.

The provision of information for older people with the condition, and for those from some ethnic minority backgrounds may need to be specifically tailored and delivered sensitively, as the myths and misconceptions about the condition may be more prevalent in these groups.

There is a variety of specific information tools especially designed for people with learning difficulties available from the national charities, as well literature and audiovisual aids to use with young children with epilepsy.

It is good practice to signpost individuals to the excellent resources provided by the epilepsy charities. The provision of information is one of the key tasks at annual review (see Appendix).

Training resources

There are training courses available from a number of the epilepsy charities, as well as from freelance epilepsy and communication trainers, on the topics included in this chapter. Details can be obtained from the charities. There are also DVD and written resources which can assist in these areas available from the epilepsy charities.

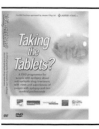

Taking the Tablets?
DVD available from all five charities listed in Box 9.2

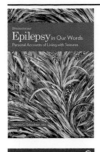

Epilepsy in our Words: Personal Accounts of Living with Seizures
(Brainstorms series)
(ed Schachter SC). Oxford University Press, 2008
ISBN 9780195330885

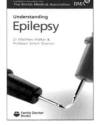

Understanding Epilepsy
Matthew Walker, Simon Shorvon
Family Doctor Books
http://familydoctor.co.uk/products/epilepsy

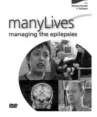

manyLives
DVD, three-disc set. Includes: interviews with key professionals in the field, oneLife, a programme of interviews with people with epilepsy talking about their condition, an epilepsy documentary and a section showing footage of real seizures. Available from Epilepsy Society.

Acknowledgements

The authors would like to thank: Judith Lanfear, Priya Bose, Susan Griffin and Sally Gomersall, who all have, or have had epilepsy, and have contributed greatly to this chapter.

References

Forsgren L, Hauser WA, Olafsson E, Sander JW, Sillanpää M, Tomson T. Mortality of epilepsy in developed countries: a review. *Epilepsia* 2005; **46** (Suppl 11): 18–27.

Hannah NJ, Black M, Sander JW, Smithson WH, Appleton R, Brown S *et al. Epilepsy – Death in the Shadows. National Clinical Sentinel Audit of Epilepsy-Related Death: Report 2002.* The Stationery Office, 2002.

Nashef L, Langan Y. Sudden death in epilepsy, in *The Treatment of Epilepsy* (eds Shorvon S, Fish D, Perruca E, Dodson WE). Blackwell Publishing, 2004.

Additional resources

Books:

Baker GA, Jacoby A (eds). *Quality of Life in Epilepsy: Beyond Seizure Counts in Assessment and Treatment.* Harwood Academic Publishers, 2000.

Cull C, Goldstein LH (eds). *The Clinical Psychologist's Handbook of Epilepsy: Assessment and Management.* Routledge, 1997.

Marshall F, Crawford PM. *Coping with Epilepsy*, 2nd edn. Sheldon Press, 2006.

Websites:

If you want to refer young people to a website for themselves, you could link to the Epilepsy Society site, www.youthhealthtalk.org/Young_people_with_epilepsy/ or an online forum www.epilepsysociety.org.uk/Forum/.

Epilepsy Charities

Brainwave The Irish Epilepsy Association; www.epilepsy.ie

The Daisy Garland; www.thedaisygarland.org.uk

DRAVET Syndrome UK; www.dravet.org.uk

Epilepsy Action (British Epilepsy Association); www.epilepsy.org.uk

Epilepsy Bereaved; www.sudep.org

Epilepsy Connections; www.epilepsyconnections.org.uk

Epilepsy HERE; www.epilepsyhere.org.uk

Epilepsy Outlook; www.epilepsyhere.org.uk

Epilepsy Research UK; www.epilepsyresearch.org.uk

Epilepsy Scotland; www.epilepsyscotland.org.uk

Epilepsy Society (The National Society for Epilepsy); www. epilepsysociety.org.uk

Epilepsy Society (Residential); www.epilepsysociety.org.uk

Epilepsy Specialist Nurses Association; www.esna-online.org.uk

Epilepsy Wales; www.epilepsy-wales.org.uk

Gravesend Epilepsy Network; www.gravesendepilepsynetwork.com

International League Against Epilepsy (British Branch); www.ilae-uk.org.uk

Matthew's Friends; www.matthewsfriends.org.uk

Meath Trust (Residential); www.meath.org.uk

Mersey Region Epilepsy Association; www.epilepsymersey.org.uk

National Centre for Young People with Epilepsy (NCYPE) (Residential); www.ncype.org.uk or

Quarriers (Residential); www.quarriers.org.uk

Scottish Epilepsy Initiative; www.scottishepilepsy.org

St. Elizabeth's Centre (Residential); www.stelizabeths.org.uk

Wales Epilepsy Research Network (WERN); www.wern.swan.ac.uk

ABC of Epilepsy, First Edition.
Edited by W. Henry Smithson and Matthew C. Walker.
© 2012 Blackwell Publishing Ltd. Published 2012 by Blackwell Publishing Ltd.

Index